W9-CCM-315

Managing the Health Care Professional

Charles R. McConnell

JONES AND BARTLETT PUBLISHERS
Sudbury, Massachusetts
BOSTON   TORONTO   LONDON   SINGAPORE

World Headquarters
Jones and Bartlett Publishers
40 Tall Pine Drive
Sudbury, MA 01776
978-443-5000
info@jbpub.com
www.jbpub.com

Jones and Bartlett Publishers Canada
2406 Nikanna Road
Mississauga, ON L5C 2W6
CANADA

Jones and Bartlett Publishers International
Barb House, Barb Mews
London W6 7PA
UK

Library of Congress Cataloging-in-Publication Data

McConnell, Charles R.
   Managing the health care professional / by Charles R. McConnell.
     p. cm.
   Includes bibliographical references and index.
   ISBN 0-7637-3130-7
     1. Health facilities—Personnel management. 2. Medical personnel. 3. Professional employees.
I. Title.

RA971.35.M28 2003
362.1'068'3—dc21

                                    2003047435

Publisher: Michael Brown
Editorial Assistant: Chambers Moore
Production Manager: Amy Rose
Associate Production Editor: Karen C. Ferreira
Associate Production Editor: Renée Sekerak
Production Assistant: Jenny L. McIsaac
Associate Marketing Manager: Joy Stark-Vancs
Manufacturing Buyer: Therese Bräuer
Cover Design: Philip Regan
Text Design, Art, and Composition: Dartmouth Publishing, Inc.
Printing and Binding: Malloy, Inc.
Cover Printing: Malloy, Inc.

Printed in the United States of America
07 06 05 04 03   10 9 8 7 6 5 4 3 2 1

Table of Contents

Preface

Managing the Health Care Professional was written with two important purposes in mind. First, it is intended as a practical guide for the first-line supervisor, middle manager, or department head who must direct the activities of health care professionals. Second, but equally important, it is meant to be a learning instrument for students of the health care professions.

Why are professionals considered as being any different from other employees? Are there not many sound reasons—as well as legal requirements—for treating all employees equally regardless of education, background, or position? It is true that in many ways professionals are the same as all other employees; they come to work each day, they experience successes and failures, they have needs as individuals, and they sometimes present problems for the manager. Nevertheless, these health care professionals are likely to be different from other employees at certain times, and in certain specific dimensions of the employment relationship.

This book identifies a number of points of departure in the handling of professional employees versus the handling of others, addressing differences in how employees approach the job, how they relate to the organization and its objectives, and how they respond to the manager's leadership.

Depending on individual circumstances, the differences between the professional and the nonprofessional may be few and barely visible, or they may be many and obvious. However, one key difference that is likely to surface in some relationships is the matter of identification. The nonprofessional ordinarily identifies with the organization; this person has a job with a particular organization. The professional, however, may feel a double identification with both organization and occupation or may even identify primarily with the occupation or the profession. This difference in identification, plus consideration of the independent nature of much professional work, provides the foundation for much of the professional employee's behavior.

Most management literature rightly stresses the critical need for uniform personnel practices and for equal and consistent treatment of all employees. Most of the literature also recognizes that every employee is unique and sometimes requires unique approaches. *Managing the Health Care Professional* proceeds a step beyond by recognizing an employee's professionalism as an important part of a mixture of characteristics that make the individual truly unique, and thus deserving of treatment that addresses that professionalism as part of the fundamental relationship between manager and employee.

CHAPTER 1

The Professional Defined: Traditionally, Legally, and Practically

*There are at least three dimensions to a profession. The width,
the height and the depth of that which may be called a
profession can be described. The three D's of a profession may
be said to be Dedication, Development, and Discipline.*

—Ted Wilson Booker

This Chapter Will:

► Review the evolution of the use of the terms *profession* (the occupation or calling) and *professional* (the person).

► Review the highlights of the portions of the Fair Labor Standards Act (FLSA) that provide a legal definition of *professional.*

► Briefly describe how the U.S. Department of Labor (DOL) administers the portions of the Fair Labor Standards Act applicable to a professional employee's designation as either exempt or nonexempt.

► Develop a practical approach toward a working definition of *professional,* especially as applicable within the health care organization.

INTRODUCTION

The *American Heritage Dictionary of the English Language* defines a profession as "an occupation or vocation requiring training in the liberal arts or the sciences and advanced study in a specialized field." The same dictionary offers three definitions of *professional,* the person. They are

1. a person following a profession;

2. one who earns his livelihood as an athlete;

3. one who has an assured competence in a particular field or occupation.

The first definition does no more than define *professional* in terms of *profession.* The second simply acknowledges present-day acceptance of the individual whose primary source of income is athletic performance as a professional of sorts. The third definition comes much closer to suggesting what *professional* means in this book. However, even this is sufficiently broad as to be frequently stretched to encompass a significant but inadequately defined proportion of the workforce.

One can find *professional* defined in literature with varying degrees of specificity depending, apparently, on the points of reference of those rendering such definitions. In his landmark work *Modern Organizations*, Amitai Etzioni referred to medicine and law as the "traditional professions." Although Etzioni also acknowledged engineering and nursing as professions, he made further distinctions relating to length of professional training, and thus suggested that "lesser professions" required less than five years of training.[1]

It is clear that many health care managers could make good use of a working definition—or at least a limited range of definitions—of *professional* that could be applied consistently through the health care organization. This chapter is intended to develop some working definitions of *professional*. Some occupations—doctor of medicine (M.D.), for example—are universally accepted as professions. Certain other occupations—such as licensed practical nurse (L.P.N.)—may not be accepted as professions by many people. Some lines must be drawn between professional and nonprofessional, and regardless of where these lines are drawn, many perceived differences remain as to whether certain occupations can indeed be considered professions. Especially concerning the regard for a given occupation, one person might think of that occupation as a profession while another thinks of it simply as a job.

Whether a person is considered a professional depends in part on a combination of at least a few objective criteria. These criteria are objective primarily in the sense that they can be counted—that is, they are either present or absent. They also include possession of an academic degree; possession of appropriate licensure, certification, or registry; and consistency with established legal definitions. However, whether a worker is considered a professional in a particular work organization can also depend on some far less tangible criteria that include the attitude and behavior of the worker, the attitude of the organization toward the worker's occupation, the worker's gender, the treatment accorded both worker and occupation by the organization, and the value structure of the organization's dominant profession.

In many respects, management of a professional is no different from the management of any other employee. Much of what the manager learns about managing the work of any employee is fully applicable to the management of the professional.

This book is confined to those areas of supervisory and management practice that sometimes—or most frequently—offer sound justification for treating the professional differently from the nonprofessional. However, much of a manager's relations with employees should not at all be influenced by whether they are professionals. Common sense, and especially principles of fair and equal treatment, should always govern a manager's relations with all employees at all times.

Attention is focused on those aspects of first-line management in which legitimate differences in style, treatment, or approach may be called for in dealing with the health care professional. Employees in every kind of working position can at times challenge the manager to come up with new approaches and unique solutions. However, even under ordinary day-to-day working circumstances and without the pressures imposed by extraordinary personnel problems, the professional may well be most effectively managed—at least in some respects—in a manner different from that applied to the nonprofessional.

The focus of this book is deliberately not on that of top management. Rather, the primary concern is the task of the lower-to-middle-level manager— whether called supervisor, department head, manager, director, head nurse, nurse manager, or comparable—of one or more groups of employees that include health care professionals. Evident throughout all of the material is a common thread that should run through any published advice for working managers: Management is getting things done through people. This approach acknowledges the fact that some employees are likely to be health care professionals, and that often these particular people are most effectively managed in a manner that recognizes, respects, and makes full use of their professionalism.

THE TRADITIONAL PROFESSIONS

The working world and the world at large have come to use the term *professional* in some extremely broad and varied ways. (In what might seem to be the extreme: "Upon examination of the crime scene," said the investigator, "I'd say this was a professional job.") Such broad uses of the term were not always the case. When great-grandmother made reference to *a professional man* (yes, the term was inherently sexist), chances are she was referring to a physician, a lawyer, or a clergyman. Even with that limited scope, great-grandmother may have gotten an argument from someone about who was or was not a professional; many people would have insisted that medicine and law were the only two legitimate professions.

These traditional definitions were rooted largely in a relationship to formal education: law and medicine were foremost among the lines of work to first limit entry to academically trained persons. The ministry remained behind; one could still become a member of the clergy without a formal, college-level education.

Although great-grandmother's reference to a professional man was indeed sexist by today's standards, it was undoubtedly rendered in all innocence. Until the latter half of the nineteenth century, the few so-called professions were almost exclusively male territory.

Today we can list many more professions than just physician, attorney, and clergyman. In truth, so many occupations are now referred to as professions that attempts to specifically define *professional* are exercises in frustration at best.

One could of course pass a law that includes a legal definition of *professional*. This is precisely what the federal government attempted to do with *professional*, and some other work-related designations, in the Fair Labor Standards Act (FLSA).

A LEGAL DEFINITION

The Fair Labor Standards Act became law on June 25, 1938. It addresses matters of minimum pay, maximum hours, equal pay, overtime pay, child labor, and record-keeping requirements applicable to most aspects of employment. The FLSA is administered by the Wage and Hour Division of the U.S. Department of Labor. The act has been amended several times since 1938, with what is probably the most important amendment being the Equal Pay Act of 1963.

Under the provisions of the FLSA, professionals are exempt from requirements governing minimum wages and overtime pay. In fact, many categories of exemptions are listed in the FLSA. However, the basic exemption from the minimum wage and overtime provisions of the act is the one most commonly referred to in speaking of exempt employees in a health care organization.

The FLSA defines a *professional employee* in a manner that says, in effect, that if an employee meets certain criteria relative to a specific job, the employee is a *professional* and is thus considered exempt from the minimum wage and overtime provisions of the act. The act also provides similar criteria for defining *executives* and *administrators*.

Minimum pay levels for professional employees are specified in the FLSA. Because these minimum pay levels, when broken down to hourly rates based on a standard work week, are higher than the prevailing minimum wage, the practical effect of being exempt is that professional employees need not be paid for overtime hours worked.

To be considered a *professional* under the FLSA, an employee in a specific position must meet the following five requirements:

1. The person must be engaged in primary duties that require

   a. advanced knowledge of the kind that must ordinarily be acquired through a course of extended study or specialized instruction, or

   b. the application of imagination or creativity, or the exercise of talent, or

   c. employment in a teaching capacity by a legally recognized educational institution.

2. The individual's work must require the exercise of discretion and judgment (references to the exercise of discretion and judgment are numerous throughout the FLSA).

3. The employee's work must be describable as primarily intellectual and varied.

4. Not more than 20 percent of the individual's time may be spent doing work that is not part of, directly related to, or performed in support of requirements 1, 2, and 3.

5. The employee must be paid not less than a specifically stated amount per week. [A rate of $280 per week became effective February 13, 1983, and this figure appeared as "current" in 2002. However, this figure is not to be taken as universally applicable, as the FLSA provides different minimum salaries applicable under differing circumstances. Up-to-date minimum salary requirements of the FLSA can be obtained through the Department Of Labor's web site (www.dol.gov).]

All interpretations of the FLSA stress the need for professional work, as defined in the foregoing requirements, to constitute the employee's primary duties. Also, under the act it is the position, not the individual and his or her qualifications, that determines the circumstances under which the person works. For example, we readily consider a registered nurse to be a professional. However, if a registered nurse chooses to change vocations and works as a payroll clerk, then that nurse is no longer considered a professional under the FLSA. Under the FLSA the professional is never defined by the individual's capability, training, experience, or licensure; rather, the person must be *employed* in a professional position to be considered a professional.

Upon cursory examination it might appear as though many persons employed by a health care organization could be defined as professionals under the FLSA . However, this is not the case because of the manner in which the requirement concerning minimum pay is applied. The requirement for the professional to be paid at least $280 per week refers to payment on a salaried basis, and not on the basis of an hourly rate. If an individual is employed, for instance, at a stated rate of $7.00 per hour ($280 for a 40-hour week), and the person's pay is calculated at that rate multiplied by the number of hours worked as recorded on a daily time record, then the employee must be considered nonexempt. To fit the definition of *professional* in the FLSA, the employee must be paid a stated salary rather than an hourly rate. In short, being salaried—and thus exempt from the minimum wage and overtime requirements of the FLSA—is, according to the definition criteria, a condition of being legally defined as a *professional* (or an *executive* or *administrator*, as separately defined in the act).

If an employee in a particular position meets all of the criteria, including salary, then that employee is a professional under the FLSA. However, numerous employees in the health care organization who do not fit the so-called legal definition still consider themselves professionals and are considered as such by their organizations. For example, few would deny that the registered nurse or the therapeutic dietician is a professional, although they may commonly be employed on the basis of an hourly wage.

Regarding the definition offered by the FLSA, we can safely say that it is not a complete test of professionalism. An employee who meets all of the definition criteria is indeed a professional, but an employee who does not meet all of the criteria may nevertheless be a professional based on other considerations.

Needless to say, the FLSA is a weighty piece of legislation because it attempts to cover virtually all wage-and-hour situations. However, several interpretive references are available as sources of information about the act and its applicability. Usually at least one such reference can be accessed through the administrative or human resources offices of most health care institutions. Three sources of FLSA information are as follows:

1. *Employment Coordinator* [formerly the *Federal Regulation of Employment Service* (FRES)], Thomson West Publishing. This multivolume reference addresses all employment practices and is updated on a regular basis. It is available both online and in hardcover.

2. *BNA Wage Hour & Leave Report*, The Bureau of National Affairs, Inc. This is a subscription service that provides biweekly reports, that facilitates tracking wage and hour topics regulated under FLSA, including overtime, minimum wage, prevailing wages, and exempt employees.

3. The official web site of the U.S. Department of Labor, *www.dol.gov*, specifically the Employment Standards Administration, Wage and Hour Division, FLSA Advisor. This site provides a great deal of useful information about wage and hour issues and includes readily accessible answers to frequently asked questions.

There is one further precaution to note when attempting to apply definitions found in the interpretive references or in the FLSA itself: some of the criteria used to define a professional are inexact and thus require a judgment call. What indeed is "intellectual and varied" work? And what requires "creativity," or how precisely can we determine the percentage of a person's time spent on "nonprofessional" work? Often when questions of legality arise, the judgment of the DOL may differ considerably from the judgment of the institution's administration, or even that of the organization's human resources department. (Although the human resources department is ordinarily the organization's primary interpreter of employment regulations, human resources practitioners sometimes find themselves at odds with the DOL's judgments.)

Department of Labor Audits and Investigations

It has been observed on many occasions that the FLSA is the one law affecting employment that is most often violated by employers. Some violations result from confusion or misinterpretation. Many employers are subject to state labor laws that often conflict with the requirements of federal law, and when state and federal law both address the same actions or circumstances the employer is obligated to comply with the more stringent of the two. However, some violations of wage and hour law result from employers' deliberately bending regulations to save money.

There is always the chance that an organization's decision to designate any particular position as professional or nonprofessional—that is, in wage payment terms, treat the position as exempt or nonexempt—will be challenged by the DOL. An audit or investigation by the DOL can occur in one of two ways: The DOL may decide to perform a routine audit of the practices of an organization selected at random; or the DOL investigators may descend upon the organization because they have received a complaint, usually from an employee. The DOL representatives will of course not reveal the source of a specific complaint, nor will they necessarily reveal whether they are there for a routine audit or because of a complaint.

A particular complaint may involve almost any aspect of wage payment, but many of the more common complaints received involve the payment (or non-payment) of overtime as determined by an employee's status as either exempt or nonexempt. In addition to the five requirements listed for defining *professional*, there are parallel requirements used for defining *executive* and *administrator*. The DOL investigators apply their judgment in comparing actual job duties with the definition criteria.

The DOL investigators may attempt to determine, for example, whether so-called "exempt" professionals are in fact treated as such in terms of how their compensation is determined. "Exempt" essentially means "salaried," that is, supposedly paid a fixed amount per time period (usually a week) regardless of hours worked. Theoretically a salaried employee is earning the same amount on any given day whether working one or two hours or remaining on the job for 12 hours or longer; a day is a day for a salaried worker regardless of how few or how many hours are worked. The salaried worker is supposedly paid not on the basis of hours worked but for doing the job. Yet some organizations have operated payroll systems that docked the pay of so-called professional workers for portions of days that were missed. For example, a dietician takes off two hours for a real-estate closing and is either docked two hours pay or is charged with two hours of vacation time. When practices such as this are in place, there is a high risk that a DOL audit or investigation will lead to a conclusion that the employee is actually being treated as nonexempt rather than exempt. Should examination of time records indicate that the dietician has consistently worked more than 40 hours per week, because the organization has tied his or her pay to time worked in one set of circumstances, the DOL may determine that the rules for nonexempt employees must apply to the dietician in all circumstances. This means that the individual should have been paid overtime—determined at one-and-a-half times the person's "regular rate"—for all hours in excess of 40 per week.

One particular practice that has caused many organizations to run afoul of the DOL involves secretarial personnel, usually those within administration or in senior secretarial positions. The practice involves reclassifying higher-level secretaries as salaried and thus exempt by raising their pay to an appropriate level (relative to the FLSA requirements) and giving them more "responsible" sounding titles. *Administrative assistant* is one such title often encountered. Doing so provides the flexibility of longer or varied hours when appropriate. Numerous organizations have made such changes apparently in the belief that the increased pay and title change were enough to justify an exempt designation. However, when the DOL applies the FLSA requirements to the jobs of such employees, these positions frequently do not measure up to the defining requirements of *administrative, executive,* or *professional* personnel, especially as concerns the "exercise of discretion and judgment" and the percentage of time spent doing various kinds of work.

When such findings result from audit or investigation, the DOL will require that for each affected person the hours worked in excess of 40 must be determined—often estimated, when specific records are not available—and that those hours must be compensated at an overtime rate. Should the DOL conclude that the avoidance of overtime payment was not intentional, the organization will be ordered to pay imputed overtime for two years past. If it is concluded that the organization was intentionally avoiding overtime payment, the payment of imputed overtime for *three* years past will be required and there could be additional legal repercussions as well.

It is therefore in the best interests of the organization to adhere to the FLSA definitions of *executive, administrative,* and *professional* employees as closely as possible in evaluating and classifying positions.

There is also a particular distinction that must always be kept in mind when classifying jobs as exempt or nonexempt. A position that fits the nonexempt definition *must* be treated as nonexempt and paid accordingly (specifically, be paid overtime for hours in excess of 40 per week). However, a position that fits the exempt definition *can* be treated as exempt (i.e., with no overtime payment), but this is not a legal requirement—at the employer's option, this position may be treated like a nonexempt position complete with overtime payment. This is precisely the case with many health care workers. For example, many registered nurses, unarguably professionals as reckoned by several different measures, are paid on the basis of an hourly rate and receive overtime pay for hours in excess of 40 per week.

Other Legal Difficulties

Rather than complaining to the DOL and waiting for an investigation, some employees choose to take legal action against employers that they believe have been evading overtime payment through various means. An increasing number of workers are demanding more from their employers. The result is a flood of lawsuits by employees, many in arguably "professional" jobs, who accuse their employers of cheating them out of overtime pay.[2]

Americans are working more hours than they have in several decades—longer than their counterparts in all other industrialized countries—and employers are trying to stretch productivity. Employers are also changing peoples' jobs and giving them hard-to-define titles that are intended to fall within the professional, administrative, or executive category. This has fueled disputes between employers and employees about the definition and responsibilities of a professional and what constitutes fair pay. In one prominent legal action in which workers contended they were owed overtime, employees claimed that although they were told they were "professionals," all important decisions were made at higher levels and they were left to simply follow orders.

During 2001, workers filed 79 federal collective-action suits against employers seeking overtime pay under the kinds of circumstances described above, surpassing for the first time class-action suits against employers for job discrimination.[2] Legal activity occurring to such an extent simply underscores the importance of the proper application of the exempt classification.

IN PRACTICAL TERMS

Many efforts aimed at defining a professional involve comparisons, comparisons among the so-called professions found in the organization as well as comparisons with supposed nonprofessionals. Several kinds of indicators can be used in defining professionals relative to each other and relative to nonprofessionals.

Comparisons among occupations may lead to some form of scale or grade assessment of professionals. However, there should be no question regarding the upper end of the professional scale; top-level professionals possess academic degrees and are licensed to practice their professions.

Most of the definition problems involve the lower end of the professional scale. Indeed, one of the basic problems is a lack of universal agreement on what actually constitutes the lower end of the professional scale. What is a profession and what is simply a job? Were one to provide a group of health care managers with a list of health-related occupations and ask these people to designate whether they considered these occupations to be professions, one would likely receive unanimous affirmation for some occupations and mixed responses for others.

To address these mixed responses, it makes sense to establish the lower boundaries of the professional scale first by looking at the applicability of the requirements of the FLSA. If a given employee is performing a given job that fits the definition of professional in the FLSA, it is reasonable to consider that person a professional. However, the FLSA does not tell us everything that we would like to know and may in fact mislead us. For example, even though the FLSA exempts professionals from overtime payment, we cannot rightly conclude that the employee who receives overtime pay cannot be considered a professional. The legislation simply states that professionals *need not* be paid overtime; it does not say that they *must not* be paid overtime. In actual practice many clearly identifiable professionals receive overtime pay, but this is done because the organization chooses to pay them overtime and is not due to a requirement imposed by law.

The lower boundary of the professional scale, and thus the difference between the professional and the nonprofessional, is often considered to be licensure, certification, or registry by some officially recognized accreditation agency or body. This is a convenient definition criterion, but because there can be many such accreditations in a health care institution, it opens up the likelihood of defining a large percentage of an organization's employees, covering all levels and all gradations in earnings, as professionals. Regardless of absolute numbers, however, one may often find that this is the fairest criterion that can be applied.

Some employees are also accorded professional status, and their positions are considered professional positions, because of the academic qualifications required of the positions held by these persons. For instance, few would argue that a graduate engineer and a graduate accountant working in their respective fields were not professionals.

Some degreed professionals may also possess some form of licensure that permits them to engage in certain practices. An engineer, qualified by degree, may go on to become a registered professional engineer (P.E.). An accountant, similarly qualified, may become a certified public accountant (C.P.A.). An individual with an advanced degree in social work may become a certified social worker (C.S.W.). These people are clearly considered professionals as long as they are employed in the activities for which they have been trained.

Entry into a particular profession may be regulated by state law. Medical degree notwithstanding, a physician cannot practice medicine without being licensed; a nurse may not practice nursing without a license; an engineer may not engage in certain practices related to public safety without a license.

Professionals may be defined at least partly by the agencies that accredit and regulate health care institutions. For instance, the Joint Commission for the Accreditation of Healthcare Organizations (JCAHO) publishes standards that call for certain positions to be filled by people with certain professional qualifications, and the health departments of the various states publish regulations requiring much the same as called for by JCAHO. Such standards and regulations have essentially the same effect: they dictate that only people with certain specific qualifications should undertake certain tasks.

An additional term to be reckoned with when considering the professional employee is *paraprofessional*. This term came into modest use throughout health care during the 1970s. *Webster's New Collegiate Dictionary* defines *paraprofessional* as "a trained aide to a professional person." This seems straightforward enough; however, arguments frequently develop as to what *trained aide* and *assists* actually mean. For example, some persons working in health care consider the registered nurse as the professional and the licensed practical nurse as the paraprofessional; others consider the licensed practical nurse as the professional and the nursing aide or assistant as the paraprofessional.

In terms of organizational requirements, one may find professional positions that the organization has said should be filled by persons who have certain qualifications. Such organization requirements (as opposed to the requirements of regulatory bodies or accrediting agencies) may occasionally include, for instance, a desire for a registered professional engineer to head a plant engineering department or a certified public accountant to run a finance division. The organization may state in its hiring criteria that these professional qualifications are required.

Treatment and behavior also have important effects, not so much on defining the professional as on determining how an employee is managed. Throughout this book it will at times be necessary to discuss some notions of professional behavior. In practice, managers come to expect certain kinds of behavior from employees who consider themselves professionals, and to some extent the professional owes the organization a certain level of professional behavior. Professionalism, however, runs a two-way course. Ideally, the employee should have a view of self as a professional and should behave accordingly, but the organization must also view the employee's occupation as a profession and should accord the employee the treatment owed to a professional.

In summary, in attempting to define a professional it is not possible to consider the employee or the position alone. Rather, it is necessary to consider the specific employee in the specific position. According to the guidelines developed in this chapter, an employee may generally be considered a professional if

- the specific employee, occupying a specific position, fits the definition of professional in the FLSA, or

- the employee has the appropriate academic degree, appropriate accreditation (licensure, certification, or registry), or both, as required by the organization, the appropriate regulatory agency, the appropriate accrediting body, or a combination of these.

A great deal of a manager's approach to an employee is governed by the organization's treatment of the professional and the employee's level of professional behavior.

Chapter 2 addresses the range of professional employees likely to be found in health care organizations and describes the kinds of qualifications that these employees are expected or required to possess.

NOTES

1. A. Etzioni, *Modern Organizations* (Englewood Cliffs, NJ: Prentice-Hall, 1964), 77–78.
2. The Associated Press, Fight for Overtime Pay Explodes in Lawsuits, *Democrat & Chronicle*, Rochester, NY, (August 3, 2002).

QUESTIONS AND ACTIVITIES

1. Do you believe it is possible for your organization to develop its own definition of "professional" and use it for determining exempt or nonexempt status for employees? If so, what restrictions must you place on this definition?

2. Offer your own explanation of the term "intellectual and varied work," supporting your explanation with at least two clear examples.

3. Exempt Worker A is salaried at $300 per week and averages 40 hours per week on the job. Exempt Worker B is also salaried at $300 per week but averages 60 hours per week on the job. Both A and B have comparable duties and equivalent levels of responsibility. An external auditor is likely to approve of one situation but not the other. Which situation is likely to be challenged, and why?

4. Describe at least two positions or occupations that you believe are clearly professional, but that do not conform to the definition of "professional" in the Fair Labor Standards Act.

5. Why can salary level alone not be used when determining whether a particular employee is exempt or nonexempt?

Professional Employees in the Health Care Organization

If the power to do hard work is not talent, it is the best possible substitute for it.
—James A. Garfield

This Chapter Will:

► Survey the proliferation and growth of professional and technical occupations in health care organizations

► Develop an illustrative hierarchy of specialized health care occupations

► Explore the apparent advantages and disadvantages of the practice of credentialing

► Identify the unique position of the health care professional in the labor market

► Offer insight into the possible future of the health professions

HISTORICAL DEVELOPMENT OF THE HEALTH PROFESSIONS

Hospitals, whether free-standing or operating as elements of health care systems, are the largest employers of health care personnel. They are also the employers of the greatest variety of occupations found in the health care setting. However, this has not always been the case. Before the twentieth century one would have been able to count all of the health professions found in hospitals on the fingers of one hand—and have unused fingers remaining.

Hospitals have not always been the sophisticated homes of healing, research, and education that we know them to be today. The word *hospital* actually contains references to the institution's early purposes. According to author Michael Crichton, hospital comes from the Latin *hospes*, which means *host* or *guest*.[1] Other sources suggest that hospital may come from the Greek *hospitium*, meaning a place for the reception of strangers and pilgrims.[2] In either case, hospital seems to have evolved directly from the same origins as *hotel*.

The first hospitals were in fact little more than hotels for the sick, where persons simply remained until they either recovered or died. Little medical care was directed toward the restoration of health. The majority of early hospitals were operated by religious orders, and what constituted medical care was provided by priests or monks and later by nuns.

Because little was known about germs and contamination and the need for cleanliness, conditions in early hospitals were grim by today's standards. Even judged by the prevailing standards of the day, hospital conditions were poor. Hospitals were not the preferred setting for one who had any choice in the matter, and for many years those persons who could afford quality care were treated at home.

For many years there were but two health professions: physician and nurse. Perhaps these early versions of physician and nurse should be referred to as occupations rather than professions, as little formal education was involved. A nurse learned nursing primarily through on-the-job training. Although some physicians studied in classes under physician–teachers, many entered the field by "reading medicine" (an apprenticeship in which one would study while observing and assisting a practicing physician).

Because physicians practiced largely in settings other than hospitals (primarily in patients' homes and private clinics), nurses represented the single health profession active primarily in the hospital setting. For hundreds of years and extending well into the nineteenth century, nurses made up 100 percent of the hospital workforce. Physicians' widespread practice in hospitals began in the mid-1800s, as the hospital concept evolved from the warehousing of the sick and dying to the restoration of health and the preservation of life.

The next two health professions to emerge were the pharmacist—or *apothecary* or *chemist*, to apply early designations—and the dentist, who emerged in the nineteenth century as more than simply a barber who also pulled teeth.

The technological progress of the past century, and especially that occurring since 1940, has been explosive. In fewer than one hundred years, dozens of specialized health care occupations have developed, and more are emerging as progress continues to accrue. Many of these new occupations have attained the status of profession.

In considering all the occupations found in a modern health care institution, personal differences may arise as to what constitutes a profession. Such differences, arising largely from individual orientation and perspective, will always exist. It is clear, however, that health care as an industry is a stronghold of professionalism. Few other industries rely as heavily as health care does on such increasingly large numbers of highly trained and specialized workers.

THE HEALTH CARE TEAM: A GENERALIZED HIERARCHY[3]

This section provides a list of the technical and professional occupations found in a medium to a large hospital. It is certainly not all-inclusive, but it is representative of the skills often found in such an institution.

Each listed occupational specialty is accompanied by a brief description of the amount of postsecondary training necessary for entry into the occupation. Also noted are the credentials ordinarily required.

The occupations are listed approximately in the order of the length of preparation time required, and their relative positions within the pay scales of health care organizations. The approximate nature of the order must be stressed for two reasons: the pay-scale relationships among the occupations do not remain the same from institution to institution, and especially from geographic area to geographic area. In addition, preparation time and credentials are in some instances different for separate entry paths into the same occupation. For example, there are three routes, each requiring a different length of time, to the registered nurse designation.

The credentials referred to in the listing are briefly defined as follows:

- *Degree* refers to academic credentials granted by an accredited educational institution, such as A.A.S. (associate in applied science, a two-year degree) or B.S. (bachelor of science, a four-year degree).

- *Diploma* refers to program completion evidence supplied by either an educational institution (for a nondegree program) or a health care institution that operates an approved school in some special field (such as a hospital school of radiological technology).

- *Certification* in most instances is accreditation by a voluntary, nongovernmental body (usually a professional society or association), upon passage of a certification examination after successful completion of a program of study.

- *Registration* in most instances is formal recognition extended by a voluntary, nongovernmental body (usually a professional society or association), upon successful completion of a program of study.

- *Licensure* is legal permission to practice a profession, extended by a governmental body (usually a state), upon passage of a licensing examination.

Many contradictions exist in how some of these credential designations are applied. What one credentialing body calls *certification* may be called *registration* by another credentialing body. Just as many other "generic" terms have varying specific applications—for example, *supervisor* and *manager* may designate different levels of responsibility within different organizations—*certification* and *registration* may or may not be applied in the same way, depending on which accrediting bodies one may be comparing.

Some contradictions extend to some of the popularly accepted designations of occupations. A case in point is provided by the varying uses of the term *registered*. A registered record administrator (R.R.A.) is registered according to the foregoing definition, but a registered nurse (R.N.) is not registered, but rather is licensed according to the definition of licensed. Similarly, a *certified* public accountant (C.P.A.) and a *registered* professional engineer (P.E.) are actually licensed.

Any voluntary accrediting body can of course refer to its credentialing process by any name that it chooses. (The sole exception is *licensure*, which is the exclusive territory of the government.) Regardless of the term applied, however:

- if recognition is extended automatically upon completion of a program, the process is *registration*;
- if recognition comes only upon passing a required, nongovernmental examination, it is *certification*;
- if recognition comes from the government as a legal right to practice, the process is *licensure*.

With the foregoing in mind, the following occupational hierarchy can be considered in proper perspective.

The Generalized Hierarchy

Physician and dentist
- From 6 or 7 to 12 or more years of combined intensive academic training and various internships and residencies. Full duration of preparation can vary markedly depending on area of concentration or specialization.
- Degree, licensure, and various certifications

Psychologist
- Six or more years of academic training, plus clinical experience
- M.S. or Ph.D. degree and licensure (in most states)

Nurse anesthetist
- Two- to four-year program, following education and licensure as a registered nurse
- Diploma, A.A.S. or B.S. degree, and certification

Pharmacist
- Five years of academic training and often one year of internship

- B.S. degree and licensure
- Pharmacists in the health care work force also include an increasing number holding advanced degrees such as M.S. in hospital pharmacy, or doctor of pharmacy (Pharm.D.)

Physician's assistant

- One- to four-year program (most common is two years) of combined classroom training and supervised practice, for persons with the equivalent of two years' undergraduate study plus appropriate experience
- Diploma or degree, certification, and licensure (in most states)
- Many physician's assistants are originally trained as registered nurses

Nurse practitioner (and nurse clinician)

- Six to 12 months of combined classroom work and clinical experience, following licensure as a registered nurse
- Diploma and certification

Biomedical engineer

- Four years of academic training
- B.S. degree
- A number of universities offer biomedical engineering as a graduate program for persons with certain technical undergraduate degrees

Dietician

- Four years of academic training and a one-year health facility internship
- B.S. degree and certification

Medical technologist

- Three years of academic training and one year of combined classroom training and clinical experience in a laboratory setting
- B.S degree and certification
- Encompasses various "technologist" positions, including chemistry, immunology, bacteriology, and hematology

Occupational therapist

- Four years of academic training and up to one year of clinical experience in the health facility setting
- B.S. degree and certification

Physical therapist

- Four years of academic training plus several months of clinical experience
- B.S. degree and certification

Registered nurse

- Programs of two years (A.A.S. degree), three years (diploma), and four years (B.S. degree), including varying clinical experience
- Diploma or degree and licensure

Registered record administrator

- Four years of academic training, usually including some work experience
- B.S. degree and registration

Social worker

- Four years of academic training
- B.S. degree
- Numerous social workers, including those earning the designation of certified social worker (C.S.W.), are educated to the level of the M.S. degree

Biomedical technician

- Two years of academic training
- A.A.S. degree

Respiratory therapist

- Two years of combined classroom education and clinical training
- A.A.S. degree and registration

Radiological technician

- Two years of combined classroom education and clinical experience in the setting of a hospital-operated school
- Diploma and registration
- An increasing number of technicians are earning A.A.S. degrees and B.S degrees in expanding educational programs in radiological technology

Nuclear medicine technician

- Up to two-year institution-based program, or one year with appropriate medical background (e.g., registered nurse, radiological technician)
- Diploma and certification

Accredited record technician
- Two-year program, often culminating in A.A.S. degree
- Diploma or A.A.S. degree and certification

Cytotechnologist
- Twelve months of training in a laboratory setting, preceded by appropriate academic courses
- Diploma and certification

Electroencephalographic technician
- Twelve months (or longer) of work-related training
- Diploma and certification

Histologic technician
- Twelve months (or longer) of work-related training
- Diploma and certification

Laboratory assistant
- One year of combined classroom education and clinical experience
- Diploma and certification
- Encompasses various "technician" positions, including electrocardiography, hematology, urinalysis, bacteriology, serology, and chemistry

Licensed practical nurse
- One- to two-year program, combined classroom education and clinical practice
- Diploma and licensure

Respiratory therapy technician
- One-year program, often institution-based
- Diploma and certification

Surgical technician
- Variety of programs, most six to 20 months in duration
- Diploma and certification

Other Professional and Technical Specialties

A number of other specialties can be found in health care organizations. Their numbers of practitioners, and perhaps even their presence, may depend on the size and character of the specific organization. Some are distinct specialties in their own right, while others are more restrictive (and thus more specialized) variations on a few occupations described earlier. A few, such as chemist and physicist, represent health care applications of broader-based professions.

These additional specialties include the following (in alphabetical order):

- Bacteriologist
- Biochemist
- Blood bank technologist
- Chemist
- Diagnostic medical sonographer
- Dosimetrist
- Hematologist
- Medical librarian
- Nutritionist
- Orthopedic technician
- Perfusionist
- Pharmacy technician
- Physical therapy assistant
- Physicist
- Psychiatric social worker
- Radiation therapy technician
- Serologist
- Speech pathologist

These lists are by no means all-inclusive. Occasionally some occupations are identified by more than one name, and new occupations develop as special interests evolve within existing occupations. As a result, new specialties split away and grow. New specialties are continually arising as new technology develops. One might go so far as to suggest that the names of some now-recognized health care occupations are foreign to many long-time health care workers. Consider, for example, whether the labels *simulation technician* and *extracorporeal technician* are readily known to all readers.

AN EXAMPLE: ONE INSTITUTION'S HIERARCHY

An illustration of an actual hierarchy of position titles was developed from the job titles used at a metropolitan, full-service teaching hospital, in the 400- to 500-bed range, employing approximately 2400 people. This institution maintained five salary scales, two of which were used in developing the list. The list was created by merging the professional and technical scale with the nursing scale; the hospital's separate scales for administrative, clerical, and service and maintenance personnel were excluded.

In developing this list, a number of professional and technical titles were deleted because they actually fell into the administrative scale. Such titles are given to persons who are working managers: Although they carry professional designations, they are considered primarily as managers in the institution's hierarchy (e.g., chief respiratory therapist).

This list approximately follows the ranking suggested in the generalized hierarchy, but includes many more positions as well. The specific institution's hierarchy is arranged in seven levels in descending order of salary grade. Except for Level 7, each of the levels represents one of the hospital's pay grades. Level 7 is an artificial level created to illustrate the relative position of "ungraded" personnel, that is, those who are employed on the basis of personal service contracts or letters of agreement. The contract or letter of agreement is common practice for two of the four skills listed in Level 7: physician and dentist. Nurse anesthetists and psychologists can be found in either category, ungraded or within a specific salary grade, depending on the institution.

The hierarchy is as follows:

Level 7

Physician

Dentist

Nurse anesthetist

Psychologist

Level 6

Nurse practitioner II

Pharmacist

Physician's assistant II

Speech pathologist

Level 5

Biomedical engineer II

Hematology technologist II

Medical social worker II

Nurse practitioner I

Physical therapist

Physician's assistant I

Psychiatric therapist II

Radiation safety technologist

Radiation therapy technologist II

Level 4

Biomedical engineer I

Blood bank technologist

Cardiovascular technologist

Clinical chemistry technologist

Clinical laboratory technologist

Cytotechnologist

Electrocardiography technologist

Electron microscopy technologist

Hematology technologist I

Medical librarian

Medical social worker I

Microbiology technologist

Psychiatric therapist I

Radiology control technologist

Radiation therapy technologist I

Registered nurse

Registered record administrator

Research associate

Respiratory therapist

Speech pathologist I

Therapeutic dietician

Ultrasound technologist

Urinalysis technologist

Level 3

Activity therapy technician

Blood bank technician

Cardiovascular technician

Clinical chemistry technician

Clinical laboratory technician

Dental hygienist

Dietary technician

Gastrointestinal technologist

Hematology technician

Histotechnologist

Licensed practical nurse II

Microbiology technician

Nuclear medicine technician

Pulmonary technician

Radiology technician

Research assistant

Respiratory technician II

Urinalysis technician

Level 2

Accredited record technician

Animal technician

Electrocardiography and electroencephalography technician

Emergency technician

Histotechnician

Intravenous nutrition technician

Laboratory assistant

Nursing technician

Operating room technician

Psychiatric technician

Respiratory therapy technician I

Level I

Dental assistant

Electrocardiography technician

Intravenous technician

Licensed practical nurse I

Pharmacy technician

Phlebotomy technician

If this list appears to breed confusion when compared with the simpler, generalized hierarchy, this is because no specific institution's hierarchy of positions ever completely aligns with accepted generic designations. Consideration of such a listing brings one into a broad area in which supposedly generic occupational names and organizational titles are hopelessly intermingled. Ask many of the technical and professional employees in a specific organization what they do for a living, and most often they will tell you what they are by citing position titles. Some occupational names are employed as position titles; however, many position titles, although not used in all institutions and perhaps unique to one institution, come to be used as occupational titles.

The listing also demonstrates how organizations make distinctions between positions that are related to each other but are somehow different in the specific hierarchy. Some examples follow:

● Technician and technologist tend to differ generically according to education and level of responsibility. Within the organization these terms may be used to differentiate hierarchical position, with technologist being the "higher" position. The technologist ordinarily has more education and perhaps different accreditation, and receives higher pay for fulfilling greater responsibility than does the technician. Consider, in the list, persons associated with hematology: the hematology technician appears in Level 3 and the hematology technologist appears in Level 4.

● "Higher" and "lower" rankings of the same title may be differentiated by the use of numerical designations or the like. Consider physician's assistant I in Level 5 and physician's assistant II in Level 6, and biomedical engineer I in Level 4 and biomedical engineer II in Level 5.

- Other terms such as "associate" or "assistant" are used to create hierarchical distinctions. Consider research associate in Level 4 and research assistant in Level 3.

In total, the hierarchy includes 75 titles. Some are variations of generic occupation titles or variations of each other, but many are substantially different from all of the others. In a larger hospital than that used in the illustration, it should not be difficult to find many more professional and technical titles. In a small institution—perhaps a rural hospital of less than 100 beds—one may find less than half the listed titles.

Whether all employees who fit into the 75 position titles are or should be considered professionals cannot be determined in any absolute sense. Any individual determination depends on the opinion of the reader and on the behavior of the worker, the organization's regard for the occupation, and the conditions of employment. Although the argument as to who is truly a professional continues, it should be clear that all titles identified in this section can fall under the broad professional and technical designation used by many health care institutions.

CREDENTIALING: PROBLEM OR SOLUTION?

Many health care organizations follow the practice of credentialing—legitimizing practitioners by way of some form of accreditation, whether certification, registration, or licensure. Persons who have worked in health care for a number of years need only compare the extent of credentialing in 1970 or even 1975 with the extent of credentialing today, in order to appreciate how the practice has spread.

Chapter 1 refers to the requirement of registration, certification, or licensure as one of the generally accepted defining characteristics of a professional. Many persons have long recognized this defining characteristic; a professional usually holds credentials of a sort. Perhaps it has been long held true that to be a professional is to be credentialed; however, recent decades have seen the logic reversed in the minds of many. Much of the present thinking is that to be credentialed is to be a professional. Some occupations appear to have made themselves into "professions" largely through the adoption of credentialing.

Current views on credentialing are broadly mixed. Some see it as a means through which positive, constructive regulation of a health occupation can be achieved. Others see credentialing as a means by which members of a given occupational group enhance their status and insulate themselves from certain risks. Professionals in a field generally see credentialing as a means of promoting quality and integrity within the field, and maintaining acceptable standards of performance. Others view credentialing as a means of restricting entry into the field, limiting or prohibiting competition, and protecting the jobs, the salaries, and the power of those actively working in the field.[4]

In recent years the practice of credentialing has been driven toward ongoing expansion by the steady growth in health care occupations. The following process has been repeated with occupation after occupation:

- Advancing technology makes health care more complex, giving rise to new needs

- To meet these new needs, new professions develop and new specialties spin off from existing professions

- New occupational specialties become more defined; practitioners organize into societies and strive to become recognized formally by means of some official designation

- Educational institutions cooperate with the professionals and create the necessary credentialing programs (which of course bring more students into the schools)

- Professionals strive for recognition of credentials as hiring criteria by health care organizations

- Members of the profession apply their status to acquire more pay and benefits, and to secure for themselves exclusive rights to do certain kinds of work

Thus professionals ordinarily enter into regulation on their own, then seek to have their credentials recognized by accrediting bodies, health care organizations, and sometimes state governments. A move toward credentialing usually begins among the members of a professional society, an organization devoted to furthering the aims and desires of workers in a given occupational field. The profession decides that it is indeed a profession and begins to seek recognition by setting up its own credentialing program. Once a program is firmly in place, the society then pressures the health care organization to hire only credentialed professionals. In many instances, the ultimate goal is to have the occupation's credentials recognized by state license and required by accrediting bodies such as the Joint Commission on Accreditation of Healthcare Organizations (JCAHO).

One need only skim the occupations listed in this chapter to obtain an appreciation of how many occupations have attained the status of professions by way of credentialing. Many health care workers are licensed, registered, or certified. Some health professionals are even subject to multiple credentials. For example, physicians, who are degreed and licensed, may also be certified, be granted specific health institution privileges, and hold medical society memberships that allow them to engage in certain activities in a given geographic area. Nurses, all of whom are credentialed by diploma or degree and state license, may hold additional credentials. Organizational credentialing already exists in a number of subspecialties. For instance, a nurse may not be allowed to work in a cardiac rehabilitation program without completing a hospital course in cardiac rehabilitation.

Professions generally begin by regulating themselves and do so with or without government cooperation. They establish the educational and entry requirements, dictate the educational programs, set rules for the practice of the profession, determine how their own members are to be disciplined, establish codes of ethics, and resist invasion by other individuals or groups.

One common criticism of credentialing is its heavy reliance on academic degrees and examinations.[5] Neither degrees nor examinations, the critics contend, necessarily ensure competence. It has indeed been established that often there is no direct relationship between examination performance and job performance.

Although credentialing is commonly promoted as a means of providing control, one often finds that most of the controls bearing on a profession are put in place by the profession itself.[6] The members of the profession establish the rules, and the rules benefit primarily the members of the profession.

As health care professions proliferate—more and more professions emerge, each more narrowly defined than the last—the practice of credentialing spreads. Some fear, perhaps with no small justification, that credentialing is fast approaching its practical limitations and that soon the fact that so many credentialed professions exist will sorely diminish the value of professional credentials. Credentials have long been regarded as something special, yet something special is no longer special if it is possessed by almost everyone.

From a management point of view, widespread credentialing has the effect of limiting economic choice. This is contrary to health care management's expressed goal of cost containment, because price competition is hampered and in some cases is prevented. The management view also holds that credentialing tends to breed territorialism: professionals may put much effort into guarding their boundaries, a practice that becomes increasingly more difficult as the proliferation of new specialties blurs the boundaries. In addition, management has long felt the pressure of being essentially forced to obtain certain kinds of help from a limited range of choices.

Restrictive credentialing tends to deepen the mystique surrounding a given profession and thus tends to elevate the self-perceived status of those working within the profession. This often causes the working professional to view the credentialed professional as somewhat more important than those without credentials, and certainly more important than management, in turn causing particular shortcomings to surface in the professional who becomes a manager (see Chapter 10).

Since the 1980s, however, voluntary sector credentialing has come under fire from a number of directions. Some professionals have experienced trouble with equal employment opportunity laws because of entry requirements; others have run afoul of antitrust laws for activities that have been seen as limiting competition. Even so, credentialing continues to flourish. However, it has become necessary for an occupation that is attempting to "go professional" by way of credentialing to proceed cautiously, and to accept the high likelihood of legal challenges to some of its rules.[7]

Even with the problems related to credentialing, the practice will not disappear. In spite of the possible hazards of more widespread credentialing, the practice will continue to spread. The best that health care managers can do is work with the requirements of the existing system and to appreciate what credentials are and what they are not. At best, credentials can be a reasonable guarantee of minimum competence in a given field. The manager must be aware that credentials cannot guarantee acceptable levels of productivity, nor can they guarantee quality results. Credentials simply indicate what a person should be able to do; in no way do they indicate what the person can or will do.

THE PROFESSIONAL AND THE LABOR MARKET

Much as any groups of persons in the labor market may be at any given time, health professionals are occasionally subject to conditions of oversupply, undersupply, and maldistribution. During conditions of oversupply—when more professionals are available in a given field than the market can absorb—salaries and benefits do not progress nearly as well as when the market is in favor of job seekers. Oversupply creates the classic buyers' market condition: there is more of a given commodity than the market can use, so the sellers (in this case, those seeking work), by their sheer numbers, keep prices low.

Although there are occasional local or regional problems, in general the health professions in the United States have yet to encounter conditions of significant or widespread oversupply. In this regard, in fact, the health professions nearly stand alone. In some parts of the country teachers, for example, have existed in a state of oversupply for considerable time. Also, occasional recessionary periods or periods of a general slowing of economic activity have triggered oversupplies of accountants and other finance professionals, human resources professionals, and several categories of engineers.

Conversely, conditions of undersupply tend to cause salaries and benefits to be inflated as organizations bid against each other for scarce skills. This represents the classic sellers' market: demand exceeds supply. In health care, however, forces are often at work to inhibit full and free competitive bidding for scarce resources. Widespread interest in controlling health care costs has been reflected in reimbursement regulations that tend to limit the amount of money flowing in to health care institutions. Such regulations have often had the effect of capping salaries at "reasonable" levels (with "reasonable" defined as a particular arm of the government may see fit to define it). However, even though true competitive bidding may not be possible, a condition of undersupply generally inflates salaries to an extent that would not be encountered were market conditions otherwise.

Within a particular city or within a given metropolitan area, a condition of undersupply frequently encourages local institutions to remain at least closely competitive with each other as far as salaries are concerned. The local pay scales for a particularly scarce skill may move in fits and starts, sporadic increments that have the effect of placing each institution in turn in a leadership position by a narrow margin. When this occurs over a period of perhaps a year or two, one is likely to find a particular skill commanding a somewhat higher average salary than skills of comparable worth to the institution, purely because of normal market forces.

Maldistribution of resources occurs when some geographic regions have more workers with a particular skill than needed, while other regions have fewer workers with those skills than required. Some regional shortages are particularly difficult to correct for health care organizations. Although certain high-skill professionals and some professional managers may be recruited from afar with all expenses paid, health care organizations are not generally known for their ability to pay interview and relocation expenses for the majority of their employees. Some institutions occasionally offer a partial payment of moving expenses as an inducement to relocate to fill a vacancy that sorely needs filling, but this is ordinarily done on an exception basis only and after all local recruiting possibilities are exhausted.

Some professionals employed in occupations that are experiencing undersupply may occasionally participate in efforts, usually loosely organized, to raise the salaries in the local area for their kind of work. Consider, for example, the experiences of one metropolitan community with several hospitals, that was subject to organized efforts in turn by pathologists, radiologists, and nurse anesthetists to increase the level of their compensation. The process consisted generally of intensive bargaining at one institution to increase the compensation, which led to the pay at that institution being used as leverage to encourage the other institutions to raise their employees' pay scales as well.

In some geographic areas and for some particular skills, institutions can count on periodic rounds of such behavior. It can also occur when one professional, either a lone operator or a member of a small department, moves to another local institution for a supposedly higher salary. Although this "bumping" might not appear particularly representative of professional behavior, to some extent it nevertheless reflects the reality of certain market forces at work. In any case, the simple existence of this practice suggests that it would be in the best interests of institutions within a region to remain in touch with each other's practices through their hospital associations and other available mechanisms (such as third-party salary surveys), and to pay realistic and competitive wages without allowing themselves to be drawn into bidding wars.

Difficult economic times can cause changes in patterns of professional employment. Nurses provided a classic example of such changing patterns during the early 1980s. In 1982 and into 1983, in many parts of the country that had experienced a shortage of nurses it became evident that shortages were easing and in places were completely disappearing. In early 1983 the American Hospital Association reported that the average hospital occupancy dropped 1.6 percent over the first nine months of 1982, and that for all of 1982 nursing vacancies dropped by as much as 80 percent. In other words, by the end of 1982, hospitals had only one fifth as many open nursing positions as they had had at the start of that year. The nursing labor pool grew as inactive nurses re-entered the field and part-time nurses secured longer working hours. Where at one time nursing may have represented a second income for some families, in the face of growing general unemployment, nursing incomes tended more and more to become the primary income for many families.

Since cost control entered the health care picture in the late 1960s, the supply of nurses has been cyclic, subject to fluctuations that have visited the industry with several periods of nursing shortages in various parts of the country. The early years of the new millennium have seen what to all appearances is the most severe nursing shortage yet. Nurses, among other staff, are a frequent layoff target at hospitals that have been financially squeezed by managed-care programs and falling reimbursements from Medicare and Medicaid. With the number of nurses on the job decreasing, those remaining have found themselves responsible for more patients and subject to longer hours, often working double shifts and mandatory overtime. These circumstances, combined with what many nurses are describing as stagnant pay and burdensome paperwork, are driving some to abandon the profession.

While the number of nurses on the job is grossly inadequate to the need, and as the number of people choosing nursing as a career decreases, the number of jobs available for registered nurses is expected to continue to increase. In late 2002 there were approximately 2.5 million R.N.s nationwide (that's four times as many nurses as physicians), and an estimated additional 450,000 R.N.s will be needed by the year 2008.

That the nursing shortage was critical during 2002 is evident in publications, such as a study released by JCAHO. The JCAHO report claimed that the lack of nurses contributed to nearly a quarter of all the unexpected problems that resulted in death or injury to hospital patients, adding to a growing body of evidence linking the shortage of nurses to ill health. As of July 2002, more than 126,000 nursing positions—that's 12 percent of the country's total nursing positions—were vacant.[8] A survey of nursing positions in New York taken during 2001 suggested that 80 percent of New York hospitals had significant nursing vacancies (while 54 percent experienced needs for nursing assistants and 34 percent were in need of various technicians and therapists), and that on average any single nursing vacancy was taking three months to fill.[9]

The average practicing hospital R.N. today is approximately 45 years of age. It is estimated that in the next ten years approximately 50 percent of the country's R.N.s will retire. At the same time, the numbers of young people choosing nursing as an occupation continues to dwindle, and experienced nurses are dropping out for the extenuating circumstance described earlier. It is estimated that, given the present (2002) circumstances, the nursing shortage, the worst the industry has seen in modern times, could take 7 to 20 years to overcome.

BALANCED BUDGETS, UNBALANCED PROFESSIONALS

A significant piece of federal legislation known as the Balanced Budget Act (BBA) of 1997 has had significant effects on several of the health professions.

The Balanced Budget Act, as the name suggests, requires that federal revenues and expenses be made to balance each year, and if they fail to balance when the budget is initially assembled, cuts must be made to bring them into balance. More than half of the total budget is immune from cuts: specifically, the defense budget, Social Security, and the interest on the national debt cannot be cut. Therefore, the cuts necessary to balance the budget have to come from the remaining portion of the budget. The largest segment eligible for cutting is Medicare, so Medicare is the target for most of the reductions mandated by the BBA.

Cuts in Medicare reimbursement to hospitals that began in 1997 have been so damaging that the amounts lost were *partially* restored in 2000. However, the same providers faced additional BBA cuts before 2000 came to an end. These Medicare cuts drove many hospitals deeply into the red, forcing occasional closures, driving additional mergers and affiliations, and leading to layoffs of nurses and other health care workers.

Some specific health care professions were directly affected by the BBA. These include physical therapists, occupational therapists, and speech-language therapists, among others. As the budget cuts impacted postacute care facilities such as skilled nursing facilities (SNFs) and home health agencies, numerous people working in these environments found themselves facing layoff. It is felt that the BBA was directly responsible for the forced closure of a number of home health agencies.

Rehabilitative outpatient services—except those provided in *hospital* outpatient divisions—were capped by the BBA's application to Medicare. In many instances the maximum number of visits or treatments that Medicare allows post-BBA is barely half of what health professionals believe many patients require for effective rehabilitation. And fewer visits or treatments means fewer such caregivers are needed. Suddenly, a number of physical therapists, physical therapy assistants, occupational therapists, speech pathologists, and others were out of work. In some parts of the country this phenomenon marked an abrupt reversal of what had been a shortage situation. For the most part, however, the health care system seems able to adjust supply and demand appropriately and redistribute resources to where they are needed— that is, in most occupational areas except nursing. With the supply of nurses nowhere near keeping up with the increase in demand, nursing will remain the troublesome area of shortage for some time to come.

Overall, however, with regard to the general labor market and when compared with other workers, the health care professional has more to sell on the market and is generally more mobile within the limits of a specific occupation (a complete discussion of mobility appears in Chapter 6).

NON-HEALTH PROFESSIONALS IN HEALTH CARE

Although the primary concern of this volume is health care professionals, and only health care professionals have been included in the listings in this chapter, certain other professionals are employed by health care organizations. These other professionals, whose skills are readily transportable across industry lines, include the following:

- Accountants, with both undergraduate and graduate degrees, some bearing the C.P.A. designation or other professional certification
- Graduate engineers, including some with the P.E. designation
- Attorneys, working as both in-house legal counsel and administrators
- Human resources professionals, both with and without various certifications

A case can be made to regard as professionals of a sort skilled tradespersons who may be employed because they possess a certain form of licensure. Various state and municipal regulations call for boiler plants to be operated by licensed stationary engineers. Certain government agencies require that some forms of electrical work and plumbing work be performed only by licensed electricians and licensed plumbers. As compared with a number of the health professions, one might develop a fairly compelling argument as to why these skilled persons should not be considered professionals. However, by requiring any such employee to be licensed, the organization is automatically extending to that employee a measure of professional recognition.

Of course any ground rules that may be applied to the management of the health care professional apply to the professional engaged in a non-health occupational specialty as well. All that may be said about the health care professional extends to the non-health professional employed by the health care organization.

THE ESSENTIAL TEAM APPROACH

Emphasis on the team approach, which is always of importance in accomplishing the work of a department, is of special concern to the manager whose group includes professional employees. The presence of professionals and nonprofessionals in the same group suggests that one manager may encounter vast differences in education, training, and background within a limited area of responsibility. Certainly there may be sufficient differences in the kinds of work the manager's employees perform. There are likely to be many differences among professionals and nonprofessionals in terms of interests and attitudes and their responses to supervision. It falls to the manager to ensure that the contributions of all these diverse individuals are pooled and effectively focused toward the care of the organization's patients.

Within the same group the manager may have a number of people who require a fair degree of operating autonomy and a number of others who may need close supervision. Indeed the manager may have within the same group the skilled professional and the entry-level unskilled worker. Given such vast differences in employees, a number of people may tend to go in their own direction and their behavior may seem to call for unique treatment.

On the one hand, the manager must be constant in handling employees, especially in regard to the organization's policies and work rules, the application of criticism and discipline, and all human relations considerations in general. Yet the manager must also manage people differently with regard to how much responsibility is placed on them and how much direct supervision is applied to them.

All employees in the department, professional and nonprofessionals alike, should have common objectives relating to the institution's patients. Regardless of this, however, these diverse individuals do not become and remain an effectively functioning team by themselves. Rather, the building of an effective departmental team depends on the manager, who must

- Set the example for all members of the group to follow, in terms of dedication to the objectives of the organization

- Help all members of the group make the best use of their individual talents

- Provide each employee with the kind of leadership that the person may specifically need

- Be ever conscious that one of a manager's most important functions is getting the efforts of a perhaps broadly diverse group of people focused on some common specific objectives

THE FUTURE OF THE HEALTH PROFESSIONS

Since the mid-1970s, essentially everyone within health care, and many in the population at large, have heard about the problems presented by the rising cost of health care. Per capita health care expenditures continue to rise, and health care continues to demand an increasingly larger share of the gross national product (GNP).

In 1950, the United States spent $12.7 billion for health care, representing 4.4 percent of GNP and at an average annual cost of $81.86 per person. In 1980, health care spending amounted to $247.2 billion, or 9.4 percent of the GNP, with per capita health care spending at $1,076.06 per year. By the end of the year 2000, the U.S. health care bill had risen to approximately $1.2 trillion, or nearly 14 percent of gross domestic product (GDP).[10] With the GDP for 2000 amounting to about $40,382 for every man, woman, and child in America, 14 percent suggests that total health care spending amounts to more than $5,000 per capita. Yet millions of people remain under-served. Compared with the 14 percent of the GDP spent by the United States, France spends 9.6 percent, Canada spends 9.5 percent, Italy spends 8.4 percent, Japan spends 7.6 percent, and Britain spends 7 percent. Yet Canadians live longer on average than Americans and Japanese live longer than both Canadians and Americans. Small wonder that so much debate rages about a health care system "that has become both unconscionably ineffective and damnably expensive."[11]

Increased health care spending and continuing medical advances suggest that more health professionals will be needed in an ever-expanding variety of specialties. Some of this growth will occur in occupations that do not exist today; some will occur in specialties that are known and regularly utilized.

An admittedly unscientific look was taken at the growth in the numbers of individuals working in 10 occupations that comprise more than three quarters of the employment in most health facilities. Listed alphabetically, these 10 occupations are administrators, dentists, dieticians, laboratory technicians, licensed practical nurses (L.P.N.s), pharmacists, physicians, radiological technicians, registered nurses (R.N.s), and technicians other than laboratory and radiological. Since approximately 1990, supplies of practitioners in nine of these fields—all except pharmacists—have increased steadily. For some fields the increases have been significant; however, for others, specifically R.N.s, the increase in supply has lagged well behind the increase in demand.

As mentioned previously, the only sampled occupation to show a net loss in total practitioners is pharmacist. Although pharmacy continues to develop as a profession of increasingly greater sophistication, the number of pharmacists has decreased, partly because of improvements in the automation of drug manufacturing. (Today's pharmacists are much less likely to be involved in compounding—the process of assembling medications from basic ingredients—than their counterparts of only a decade earlier.) Also, because there is a shortage of pharmacists in some parts of the country, some pharmacists, as for many nurses, are reacting negatively to an increasingly hectic pace and increased paperwork. In the second quarter of 2002, it was estimated that nationwide there were more than 7000 openings for retail pharmacists alone, plus an uncounted number of pharmacy openings in the institutional setting (primarily hospitals).[12]

Yet the general population continues to expand and thus the need for health services continues to grow, and the numbers of people entering the majority of health occupations continue to grow—although, as noted above concerning registered nurses, for some occupations the growth is insufficient to meet the expanding demand. Nevertheless, one may be reasonably safe in assuming that the majority of health professions can still be considered growth occupations. More professionals will enter the workforce as new specialties develop, and more professionals will enter health care organizations as existing specialties grow more complex and sophisticated and continue to become more professionalized. In the coming years the health care manager can expect professional employees to increase as a proportion of the organization's total employment. Some managers who today supervise no professional employees are likely, in the future, to find themselves supervising a mix of professional and nonprofessional employees.

NOTES

1. M. Crichton, *Five Patients* (New York: Alfred A. Knopf, Inc., 1970).

2. C. V. Letourneau, History of Hospitals, Part I, *Hospital Management* (March 1959): 8.

3. The generalized hierarchy was developed using as a primary guide the *Allied Health Education Directory*, 9th ed. (Monroe, WI: American Medical Association, 1987). Directory information was updated and supplemented with information from various schools and programs.

4. N. Weisfeld and D. Falk, Professional Credentials Required, *Hospitals* (February 1, 1983): 74–79.

5. Ibid.

6. Ibid.

7. Ibid.

8. The New York Times, Patient Deaths Linked to Lack of Nurses, *Democrat & Chronicle*, (August 8, 2002).

9. B. Avallone, Hospitals Want Medicaid to Help Pay Nurses More. Albany Bureau, *Democrat & Chronicle* (January 13, 2001).

10. The term "gross national product" (GNP) has largely been replaced by "gross domestic product" (GDP) as being more descriptive of the total value of the goods and services produced by the U.S. economy.

11. R. Reno, U.S. Health Care System is a Big Loser. *Democrat & Chronicle* (June 4, 2002).

12. Staff and wire reports, Pharmacists' Jobs Unfilled. *Democrat & Chronicle* (April 2, 2002).

QUESTIONS AND ACTIVITIES

1. Select two occupations from "The Generalized Hierarchy" and describe their origins. Explain how and why you believe they developed as they did.

2. Explain why it is impractical to attempt to utilize universally applicable definitions of certification, registration, and licensure, and provide examples to support your explanation.

QUESTIONS AND ACTIVITIES *(continued)*

3. Describe the fundamental differences between and among the three routes to the designation of registered nurse (R.N.): associate's degree, diploma, and bachelor's degree. Indicate what you believe to be the primary strength of each route.

4. Compare and contrast the terms "technician" and "technologist," providing two comparative examples and describing the apparent differences between the two levels.

5. Select two health care occupations that require licensure, certification, or registration, and trace their evolution from beginning to the status of profession.

6. Identify what you believe to be the most significant shortcomings of credentialing, if any, and describe their effects in detail.

7. Does credentialing ever display any specific economics effects? If so, what are these effects and what are their implications in the labor market?

8. Describe in detail what you believe occurs when multiple institutions operating in the same geographic area get into "bidding wars" for the services of scarce professionals.

9. Describe how you would approach recruiting as a scarce skill, so as to bring more practitioners into your geographic area.

10. Explain why it could conceivably require "7 to 20 years" to reverse the shortage of registered nurses.

11. If the population and its health care needs are continually expanding, how do you explain the fact that employment in some health occupations is decreasing?

12. Using examples, describe in detail the apparent differences between a "professional" and a "skilled trade practitioner."

13. Taking management's point of view, describe in detail two major undesirable effects of what was described as "salary bumping."

14. Pick one occupation that you can assume is in short supply in your geographic area, and develop a multistep plan for bringing more of its practitioners into the area.

15. Explain why labor shortages appear to occur in cycles, and describe the apparent phases of such cycles.

CHAPTER 3

From School to the Real World

The things taught in schools and colleges are not an education,
but the means of an education.
— Ralph Waldo Emerson

This Chapter Will:

► Explore the principal problems encountered by the professional in making the transition from school to the work organization.

► Examine the problems resulting from the mismatch of the new professional employee's expectations with the organization's expectations.

► Delineate the role of the department manager in helping the newly hired professional successfully adapt to the health care organization.

A GAP BETWEEN EDUCATION AND WORK

In the process of obtaining their formal education, students pursuing the health care professions, or for that matter many other disciplines, acquire both skills and expectations. The objective of any program of study is to impart specific knowledge and skill to the students. All programs of professional study, whether carried on in the university, the community college, the trade or technical school, or the health care institution itself, focus on this common objective.

In most instances the objective of providing the student with knowledge and skill is well served. However, during the process of learning the student is experiencing some degree of indoctrination into the ranks of the occupation or profession, and is absorbing some of the mystique of that particular line of work. This process leads to the formation of expectations—sometimes lofty expectations, especially in the newly trained professional who has not yet experienced organizational life in the health care setting. These expectations may eventually lead to a clash between the new professional's preparation and the reality of the working world.

Professionals who have recently graduated from school bring to the health care organizations both their skills and their expectations. These professionals and their employing organizations are usually quick to recognize that their job performance is directly influenced by skills and abilities acquired during the educational process. However, neither employee nor employer is nearly as quick to recognize that job performance is also strongly influenced by expectations. When expectations formed in school are not immediately met on the job, problems that at times seem insurmountable can—and often do—result.

Many postsecondary programs, especially programs of professional study, are presented with an understandable bias. Chances are the individual student believes that the profession being studied is truly important; otherwise, he or she might well not be there. The belief in the importance of the profession may be held even more strongly by instructors who have chosen to devote themselves wholly to learning and teaching in that particular field. Most students who have attended postsecondary education have undoubtedly encountered teachers who have been so immersed in their subjects that each seems to project the belief that this particular subject is surely more important than all others. Through repeated exposure some students begin to acquire some of the teacher's projected belief in the "exceptional" nature of the field.

Another consideration is that with much of the education occurring in a purely academic setting, the student is initially oriented to the profession in a relatively pure sense, uncolored by the realities of application. The gap between theory and practice remains unbridged. Theory is, of course, required as foundational for the learning of any profession. However, theory remains only theory until it is put into practice. Even hands-on educational activities and participative activities, such as case studies and exercises, lack some vital connections with reality, such as an individual's emotional involvement in an actual situation, and often the risks inherent in the situation. Addressing a problem presented as a case study, and making a decision that has no actual consequences, is hardly the same as addressing that problem for real. In reality, making a decision can affect someone's employment or health, and can cause monetary expenditures or losses. Essentially every decision made in the workplace involves two characteristics that are absent in the classroom: uncertainty and risk. Any decision of consequence involves some uncertainty; there are no guarantees that the chosen course of action is absolutely the right one. And in any decision of consequence something is always at risk, as there are costs associated with being "wrong."

Indeed, because education is not application—regardless of how much effort is put into making the education practical—the gap between theory and practice remains unbridgeable until the student graduates, begins work, and makes the connection between the two. The principal problem lies in the fact that many students emerge from their programs unaware, or only vaguely aware, of such a gap. The educational programs generally instill a strong sense of what *should be* but rarely communicate a full appreciation of what *is*.

Once in the working world, newly graduated professionals begin to experience conflicts among their notions of how the profession should be pursued, how it is actually pursued in practice, and even how it may be pursued in a particular organizational setting. Many nurses, for instance, go through nursing school with unflagging dedication and enthusiasm, only to discover that hospital nursing is not all that they thought it would be. Said one nurse who admits she came close to abandoning hospital nursing during her first year: "I know now that I expected it to be something entirely different. All my life I had this mental picture of a starched-white-uniformed Florence Nightingale quietly and efficiently bustling from patient to patient. I know that things were said about problems—shift rotation, weekend work, demanding physicians, and troubles with management—but none of this really sank in until I was there and had to put up with it."

Newly graduated professionals, quite understandably, enter the organization with a limited sense of commitment. They do not yet fully share the goals and objectives of this specific organization. However, their expectations of the profession and their belief in the contributions they are prepared to make are high. For a great deal of the early employment relationship, new professionals see themselves as giving in full but may not yet see the organization as providing all the conditions that were supposed to be there.

The first few months in the work organization are critical for the newly graduated professional. During this period the new professional is highly likely to become discontented if all the acquired expectations, so subtly planted, nurtured, and reinforced in school, are not met.

A MISMATCH OF EXPECTATIONS

The discussion thus far has focused on the expectations of the newly graduated professional. However, the organization has expectations of the professional as well, and often these do not agree with the expectations of the new employee. Consider, for example, registered nurses. Registered nurses enter the health care workforce by way of bachelor's degree programs, associate's degree programs, and diploma programs. (The diploma programs, generally three years combining classroom work with clinical experience, are steadily decreasing in number.) Because of how they were educated, nurses from the three kinds of programs may well enter the health care workforce with different levels of expectations. Once in a hospital, however, all may find that the hospital organization expects them to perform the same tasks in the same manner. Because their expectations are different, some may feel satisfied and challenged, some may feel that they are in over their heads, and some may feel frustrated and bored. Thus some nurses, particularly those with bachelor's degrees, may actively seek relief from what they refer to as non-nursing tasks. These nurses experience further frustration when they begin to realize that certain other nurses, and perhaps the organization itself, see these non-nursing tasks as elements of traditional bedside nursing.

This is not to suggest that either set of expectations—that of the individual or that of the organization—is incorrect. In truth, when there is a mismatch of expectations between professional and organization, often both sets of expectations are well off-center. If the newly graduated professional's expectations seem unrealistic, the organization's are equally unrealistic. Yet if a potential mismatch of expectations is not taken into account when a new professional first joins the organization, the resulting situation can lead to a disillusioned employee and a disappointed organization.

Numerous examples of mismatched, unrealistic expectations of both employee and organization are evident from the experiences of holders of the master of business administration degree (M.B.A.) and the master of hospital administration degree (M.H.A.). Many new M.B.A and M.H.A. graduates leave school enthused and generally charged up, expecting to immediately be given the helm of an organization, or at least a substantial organizational unit. Nearly as many are immediately crushed when they find themselves in advisory, staff, assistant-to, or what are essentially "gofer" positions. On the other hand an occasional organization may expect the new M.B.A. or M.H.A. graduate—particularly if his or her degree was granted by a "name" school (such as Harvard or Stanford)—to be the savior who can walk in, take charge, and immediately turn things around.

The final three decades of the twentieth century saw widespread growth in the numbers of master's degree programs. Many schools launched new M.B.A. programs, and many added graduate programs in health services administration, creating what in some respects has been an oversupply of master's-prepared individuals seeking employment in administrative roles in health care. Many students thus prepared left school with high expectations of immediate employment in significant positions. These expectations immediately collided with the realities of a saturated supply of new graduates and a market unable to absorb all of them.

THE ORGANIZATION'S ROLE

The organization has two key functions, one general and one specific, in dealing with real and potential mismatches of expectations. The general function consists of establishing working relations with professional schools and their programs. The specific function consists of helping each new employee to adapt to the organization.

Professional Education

The organization can help shape the expectations of new professionals in the educational process by active involvement with the schools and their programs. In this respect, health care organizations have long had a considerable edge over other kinds of organizations, because educational experiences such as internships and work experience programs have been in place for years. Health care organizations have long made use of *doing* as one of the surest learning processes.

It is not enough simply to make internships and work experience programs available. The health care organization has a responsibility to work closely with schools as they develop their programs, and to keep persons in academia abreast of the needs in the organizations that employ these schools' graduates. Generally, the closer the organization can be brought to academia, the narrower the range of conflict between the new professional's expectations and the expectations of the organization.

The Newly Hired Professional

Those who are responsible for recruiting and placing the new professional should act early to instill in the new hire an honest, realistic view of the organization. The new hire immediately becomes one of the work group, and falls under the influence of his or her coworkers. It is rare that all employees in a group, especially a group of any appreciable size, completely share the same attitudes and outlook. Should the organization's practice be to pair a new employee with a veteran employee for purposes of orientation, the manager would do well to choose the veteran whose attitude and level of cooperation are exhibited in the kinds of behavior desired of the new employee. In other words the manager can set the stage for success or failure with the new employee simply by teaming that employee with the right or wrong person. Place the new hire under the wing of a frustrated, complaining employee and the result is likely to be another frustrated, complaining employee. Place the new hire in the care of a valued performer, though, and the chances of developing another valued performer are increased.

In bringing the new professional on board, the organization, through its human resources division and its first-line managers, should

- provide to educational centers thoroughly realistic recruiting information, and not oversell the organization as absolutely the ideal place to work, located in the ideal community. Although the health care organization's undoubtedly noble objectives can be stated in a straightforward manner, it is misleading to convey the picture of one's organization as the undisputed health care Mecca of a significant part of the world. Be open about the tangible specifics of employment such as pay scales, benefits, and work schedules, and be as willing to tell potential candidates what the organization does not have as well as what it does. A recruiting presentation should indeed be a sales pitch, but as for a sales pitch for a manufactured product by a principled salesperson, the pitch should be an honest attempt to sell the organization, and perhaps the community, on its merits and leave potential employees with a clear idea of what to expect.

- conduct thorough, honest interviews. Interviews, as much as recruiting presentations, should provide an opportunity for the job candidate to obtain as clear a picture as possible of the organization, the department, and the specific position. Even though the organization may be keenly interested in filling a particular position, an interview should never be assumed to be a one-way transfer of information. Professionals require, on average, more selling or convincing; frequently they have more employment options than unskilled or semiskilled workers. Indeed, many upper- and middle-level professionals are often in effect interviewing the organization while the organization is interviewing them. All rules of thorough, nondirective interviewing should come into play when interviewing the professional. The candidate should be given every opportunity to ask questions about the organization as well, and is entitled to straight answers.

- provide thorough, meaningful orientation. Although the human resources department may routinely conduct general orientation sessions for all new employees, the largest part of a new professional's orientation should be attended to by the department manager and should include the following:

  - Information about the organization's plans and its goals for the future and the status of the organization, both financial and otherwise

  - Information on career ladders, delineating the various upward moves potentially available to the employee if earned through performance

  - Full orientation to employee benefits programs and thorough familiarization with policies and other programs (such as tuition assistance) that have a bearing on professional growth and development

  - Complete familiarization with the building and grounds, especially with the locations of key departments

  - Thorough grounding in the specific procedures for performing the appropriate kind of professional work as it is expected to be performed within the department

Much of the process of properly bringing a new professional into the organization lies in the hands of the department manager. The manager must teach, guide, and acquaint the employee with the organization and its people, and with the interrelationships among organizational units. The manager should approach each new employee with as much attention and concern as would be given to a major new project. Indeed, each new employee, professional or otherwise, is a major new project for the manager.

The manager of professional employees must be keenly aware of the high likelihood of conflicts in expectations. The manager bears a major responsibility in successfully bringing the new professional into the organization. How well the new professional bridges the gap between school and the organization, between theory and practice, and between expectations and reality depends largely on the efforts of the manager.

QUESTIONS AND ACTIVITIES

1. Do you believe that opportunities for continuing education and development are often more important to professionals than to other employees? Why or why not?

2. Using the concepts of risk and uncertainty, thoroughly explain why classroom experience can never fully simulate situations that will be encountered in the work setting.

3. Do you believe that an incoming employee's job performance can be influenced by that person's expectations? Why or why not, and how might such influence be experienced?

4. Provide at least two detailed examples of instances in which there are noticeable differences between what one expects as a student and later encounters as an employee.

5. Fully describe the value of mentoring in introducing a new professional employee into the work organization.

6. Describe at least three approaches that can be applied to help minimize the clash of expectations between the new professional and the organization.

7. Explain why the professional employee may often form a stronger commitment to the occupation or profession than to the work organization.

QUESTIONS AND ACTIVITIES *(continued)*

8. Describe the role of the department manager in the orientation of the new professional employee, and describe how the manager can help minimize the potential mismatch of individual and organizational expectations.

9. Explain in detail how an individual might acquire unrealistic expectations before entering the work organization, and describe the results commonly encountered when such expectations are not borne out.

10. How would you define, describe, or explain the "mystique" of an occupation or profession?

CHAPTER 4

The Professional and the Nonprofessional: Where Is the Line?

How important is your job?

It is told that in ancient Greece, some politicians decided to downgrade one of their number, and so got him appointed Public Scavenger. But he fooled them. He set out to show one and all what could be done with such a humble assignment.

He wiped out unsanitary conditions, promoted civic cleanliness, stimulated civic pride. It turned out, after a few years, that the post of Public Scavenger became one of considerable honor and responsibility—sought by the best of men.

A job is what you put into it.

— Jacob M. Braude, *Lifetime Speaker's Encyclopedia*

This Chapter Will:

► Establish a rationale for the fair and reasonable comparison of professional and nonprofessional employees.

► Identify and highlight the factors that may distinguish the professional from the nonprofessional employee.

► Explore, from the perspective of the manager, the implications of the task of maintaining equivalent relationships within a group composed of both professionals and nonprofessionals.

THE HAZARDS OF COMPARISON

The brief tale of the public scavenger was related to establish part of the foundation for the discussion that follows: a job is indeed what the worker makes of it. There is no intent to suggest even remotely that professionals are somehow better or more important than nonprofessionals; clearly they are no better than other employees, and their importance, as indeed is the case for all workers, is relative to the needs to which their talents and efforts are applied. Also, it would be futile to attempt to establish professionals as more important than others given the variety of possible definitions of *professional* and the inevitable controversies as to what occupations are professions. The discussion is pertinent only if accompanied by the assumption that every occupation is of value to the health care organization, and every employee is a potentially valuable contributor to the fulfillment of the organization's objectives.

If all employees put forth maximum effort to make the most of their jobs, a troublesome collection of variables is eliminated and the differences between professionals and nonprofessionals are more apparent. However, people vary considerably in what they put into their jobs. Given the variations in the relationships between people and their positions, it is impossible to suggest to the manager a particular style or approach that always works with an employee of a particular occupational level. Rather, it can be suggested only that a situational management style is called for in supervising a group that includes people with a variety of educational levels, personalities, and attitudes. Each personal contact a manager has with an employee represents a potentially different situation, and each manager's style must adapt accordingly.

It is difficult at best to make comparisons between the professional and the nonprofessional, as the terms *professional* and *nonprofessional* do not represent absolute entities that exhibit their own sets of unvarying characteristics. Instead, the two terms are more appropriately described as representing broad concepts rather than precise designations. Because a professional may be defined by an individual's attitude and behavior within a given work setting, taken in conjunction with a limited number of objective criteria, one must deal to a considerable extent with generalizations.

Generalizations are not without inherent problems. G. K. Chesterton is quoted as saying, "All generalizations are dangerous, including this one." Some generalizations are necessary, though, so that one can differentiate between professional and nonprofessional for the purpose of assessing management style for employees of differing occupations. This practice is acceptable if one remains aware of the hazards of generalization, and proceeds with the knowledge that no conclusions arising from broad generalizations can be considered constant, immutable truth. It is best to think of the points of comparison for the professional and nonprofessional as indications of tendencies and inclinations that may be borne out in the long run, knowing that they often may be inappropriate in individual cases.

In pursuing comparison of the professional with the nonprofessional, it is necessary to limit one's consideration to the factors that can vary from person to person. That is, an appropriate comparison of a particular professional employee with a particular nonprofessional employee is most reliably undertaken if

- both have approximately the same amount of work experience;

- both possess approximately the same amount of knowledge of the organization and equal familiarity with its workings;

- both are equally willing and able to fulfill the requirements of their positions; and

- both fulfill a necessary role in helping the organization achieve its objectives.

The only absolute, objective differences between the professional and the nonprofessional are professional education and appropriate accreditation. However, these differences are superficial and provide no true basis for differentiation between the two. The presence (or absence) of professional credentials does not dictate whether a particular employee should be managed in a manner different from other employees. Rather, a blend of individual attitude and behavior, combined with one's approach to their occupation and their relationship with the organization, begins to suggest the basis for comparison. Based on such less-than-objective considerations, one can begin to describe how a professional might—or perhaps should—differ from a nonprofessional.

Consider these simple examples. With all factors other than qualifications and behavior held equal according to these precautions, a department manager may draw valid conclusions from the comparison between

- a registered nurse and a nursing assistant who have both worked on the same unit long enough to be completely oriented;

- a therapeutic dietician and a diet clerk who are likewise fully oriented to their positions, and

- a registered record administrator and a medical record clerk who are long-time employees of the same department.

All valid comparisons of professional and nonprofessional must also assume the presence of an acceptable degree of professional competence. This must be demonstrated competence, not simply the possession of the appropriate credentials. Indeed, it has frequently been proven that possession of the appropriate education and accreditation is no guarantee of professional competence. Meaningful comparison must also assume a reasonable level of professional behavior, as will be discussed in Chapter 5.

LOOKING FOR DISTINCTIONS

There are dimensions of working relationships for which the general tendencies of professionals and those of nonprofessionals are often differentiated. Treated here in a brief overview, most of these are taken up at greater length in subsequent chapters.

Directness of Supervision Required

The professional employee should require less direct supervision than the nonprofessional does in the pursuit of day-to-day activities. To perform a task, an employee must know a number of things about that task: what to do, how to do it, when it must be done, the results that are expected, and ideally, why the task must be performed. The professional should require less attention from the manager concerning the what, how, when, and why of a task. In directing the professional, the manager should be able to focus on the expected results and leave much of the rest to the employee. Once the expected results are known, the professional should be able to exercise considerable control over the total process of achieving those results. The nonprofessional generally requires more managerial attention to the individual processes. In short, the professional is generally capable of a greater amount of self-management, especially in matters concerning how tasks are performed.

Independence of Judgment

A professional should be expected to display more independent judgment than the nonprofessional. Recall, from the discussion of the Fair Labor Standards Act and the definition of a professional, the frequent references to the exercise of discretion and judgment. The exercise of discretion and judgment is fully consistent with the lesser degree of direct supervision that should be required: The nonprofessional's focus may be primarily on doing, whereas the professional's focus may be more on what to do and how to do it. Indeed, a major part of the rationale for paying the professional more than the nonprofessional lies in the organization's expectations that the professional exercises a greater degree of discretion and judgment.

Degree of Responsibility and Accountability

The professional is generally considered more responsible and accountable for task performance. This is, of course, related to directness of supervision and the need for individual judgment. There are trade-offs, though. In supervising the professional, the manager often gives up a considerable measure of direct control in exchange for the professional's higher level of responsibility and accountability. In the process of giving up some measure of supervisory control, the manager surrenders the authority for task performance. However, the manager *gains* more operating freedom by not having to exercise direct control over the employee's every move.

This is delegation in its purest and simplest form: the manager surrenders task performance authority and holds the employee responsible for that performance. The manager of course remains responsible to higher authority for the professional's task performance, but if the delegation is thorough in every respect the professional is functioning as a direct extension of the manager. The concept of complete delegation is extremely important in the relationship between the manager and the professional employee. Through delegation of task performance authority, the professional is allowed to perform as a department of one, responsible to the manager, while the manager's attention is focused on legitimate day-to-day concerns.

Degree of Self-Motivation

Each individual is driven by a unique mix of needs. The professional is much more likely to be subject to a more compelling mix of needs, most likely the same needs that prompted the individual to seek a profession in the first place, as opposed to simply looking for a job. Indeed the fact that certain high-skill professionals go through such prolonged periods of work and study to enter their professions should give weight to the claim that many professionals are highly motivated individuals.

It is also common for an employee to display a high level of motivation derived at least in part from a strong sense of identification with an organization. Health care workers in general serve the organization and its patients as well as serving themselves. The working professional is often serving the *profession* as well. To list additional drives that can come into play, the professional may

- more strongly desire to achieve growth within the organization or the profession, or to earn larger amounts of money;

- be driven by a generally stronger need for individual accomplishment;

- be more dedicated to the aims of his or her own occupation (the profession);

- harbor a strong liking for the work itself; and
- have a strong need for occupational security that can be more completely met by a profession than by a job.

As compared with the nonprofessional, the professional is much more likely to be working toward the fulfillment of needs that are largely psychological. To the professional, the need for accomplishment and fulfillment is often stronger than it is for the nonprofessional. Becoming a professional is to many people the way in which to achieve fulfillment of one's psychological needs through work.

Orientation to Growth

In general, the professional is most likely to strive for learning and growth within a constantly changing health care environment, and especially within a constantly changing occupation. Borrowing some consideration from thoughts about human motivation, it can be suggested that many of the same drives that cause a person to seek a profession in the first place also prompt that person, as a practicing professional, to become oriented toward growth. A strong growth orientation may derive from a combination of previously considered factors:

- An individual dedication to the profession,
- A strong liking of the work, to the extent of wishing to do more of it and do it better
- A search for increasing levels of accomplishment, keeping the individual moving toward increasingly challenging tasks

Division of Loyalty

The professional is likely to experience more in the way of divided loyalty than is the nonprofessional. Partly because the professional is more mobile, and partly because of a likely degree of dedication to one's profession, the professional, although perhaps loyal to the organization, may be equally or even more strongly loyal to the profession.

In regard to the combination of mobility and loyalty, one's line of work is more likely to carry the professional to another organization. The profession may come to mean a great deal more than just the specific position in one particular organization. This is not ordinarily so for the nonprofessional, who is considerably less likely to change organizations for the sake of an occupation but may be quicker to move to another organization because of factors that are not inherent in the work, such as job security, pay and other benefits, or more humane treatment. A professional generally attaches to an organization if it supplies what he or she expects of it. However, when put to the test, the professional is much more likely than the nonprofessional to place loyalty to occupation before loyalty to organization.

Extent of Job Mobility

As suggested, the professional generally enjoys more freedom to move from organization to organization. Simply put, the professional has more portable skills. The nonprofessional employee is far more likely to make a change of occupation in order to remain with the same organization, whereas the professional is more likely to change organizations in order to remain in the same line of work. A professional has skills that are more likely to be in demand in a number of organizations. The professional's credentials often constitute an eminently salable commodity, and as a result the professional has more opportunity for ready movement to other organizations.

FROM THE MANAGER'S PERSPECTIVE

The management of the health care professional usually requires a more refined level of practice of certain basic supervisory skills. It certainly requires more subtlety and finesse. Successful management of the health care professional also requires emphasis on consultative and participative leadership styles. On the plus side, or at least what may seem to be the plus side to managers who have truly mastered the art of delegation, managing the professional requires far less hand-holding and specific task guidance than managing the nonprofessional.

Ordinarily, the professional employee cannot, and should not, be dealt with in the same manner as other employees. This is so, however, not because of any basic human differences but rather because of the kinds of work that professionals do, and the manner in which they relate to that work.

In many ways, it is always important for the manager to regard all employees fairly and equally, and it is essential that the manager apply the organization's rules and policies equally to all employees. Regardless of a person's level of education and their occupation, the manager must forever consider the employee as a whole person and not simply as a piece of animated production equipment. Every employee should be allowed the opportunity to experience a manager-to-employee relationship based on dignity and respect. However, equal respect and regard do not necessarily mean equal supervisory treatment in all aspects of the employment relationship. There have been, and always will be, some employees who need more of the manager's attention than others.

The professional employee may often require a looser, more open style of supervision than the nonprofessional. But the presence of several levels of both professional and nonprofessional employees in the department, a condition often encountered in health care organizations, may give rise to the question, Can a manager successfully supervise such a mixed group? The answer is of course affirmative. It is found in a flexible, adaptive leadership style reflecting the manager's belief that every employee is different, but special, and the manager's focusing on establishing and maintaining a strong one-to-one relationship with each person in the work group.

Regardless of an individual's background or skills, the manager must concentrate on nurturing the vital manager-to-employee relationship that serves the person's unique needs while making best use of the employee's capabilities. If a sound relationship exists with each and every employee, the manager is likely to be acting out a belief in fair and equal treatment for all. As long as the manager handles the differences in supervision based on each employee's occupation, then all interactions will appropriately occur within the context of those one-to-one relationships.

One of the best—albeit one of the most general—pieces of advice that can be given to the supervisor is to *know the employees*. To this, one may attach an additional consideration: Although it is never too late to begin improving the relationship with any particular employee, the best time for creating the foundation for a sound one-to-one relationship is when the employee is new to the organization. The manager would do well to devote as much time to a new employee as to a new major assignment. Indeed, each new employee *is* a new major assignment for the manager.

Know the employees, and know them well. Some of them need more or less regular contact than others. Some require reassurance at regular intervals; some function for considerably longer periods without reassurance. Although all may be deserving of praise when praise would appear to be warranted, only some of them need frequent praise to keep them going. Some may accept constructive criticism squarely, straight from the shoulder; some may need to be approached more tactfully when criticism is deserved.

The manager might often feel frustrated by the discovery that there is no standard formula for dealing with employees. However, even in a work situation that is sympathetic to the manager and that fosters appreciation of the manager's task, it is necessary to recognize that differences among employees go with the territory. There is no single "correct" way of dealing with people. Each person is an individual and must be dealt with as such. A manager with 10 employees may discover on any given day that there are 10 "correct" ways of dealing with people, regardless of whether they are professional or nonprofessional.

LOOKING FOR THE LINE

This chapter's title was intended to encourage consideration of the perceived dividing line between professional and nonprofessional employees in the modern health care organization. Where, indeed, is the dividing line between professional and nonprofessional? It is suggested that if at chapter's end one is left with the impression that the dividing line is at best hazy and at worst nonexistent, one is probably on the right track.

It is of course relatively simple to compare any two jobs or occupations using the several dimensions or characteristics briefly introduced earlier in the chapter, specifically:

- Extent of supervision required (direct or indirect; close or loose; and so on)
- Independence of judgment required of the person doing the job
- Degree of self-motivation sustaining one in the occupation
- An employee's orientation and attitude toward growth and development
- The preponderance of an employee's likely loyalty toward either the organization or the occupation
- The relative ease with which one might move across organizational lines while remaining in the occupation in question

If these criteria were all that determined professionalism or the lack thereof, it would not be too difficult to set some arbitrary but reasonable limits and sort most of an organization's positions into two categories: professional and nonprofessional. The task might be rendered all the easier by also factoring in the presence or absence of licensure, certification, or registration. Yet all of these considerations will not always determine what, for all practical purposes, may be considered a profession and what is decidedly not a profession. There is another essential element to consider.

The anecdote that opened this chapter—the tale of the public scavenger—concluded that in the end, a job is what one puts into it. In addition, to a considerable extent a job is also what the *organization* puts into it. These two sides of what frequently seems to be a decidedly unbalanced coin represent an important area addressed in the following chapter, "Professional Behavior and Professional Treatment."

QUESTIONS AND ACTIVITIES

1. Fully explain why it is reasonable to assume that the typical professional employee should require less direct supervision than the typical nonprofessional.

2. Identify and describe the differences between *responsibility* and *accountability* as they apply to both professional and nonprofessional employees.

3. From the perspective of the department manager, identify and describe both the benefits and the risks inherent in surrendering task performance authority to employees and giving up a measure of direct control over those employees.

4. Describe the essential differences between the consultative and participative styles of leadership, and for each style provide a description of its hypothetical application in a manager's relationship with a professional employee.

5. If it is true that "the only absolute, objective differences between professional and nonprofessional are professional education and accreditation," how do other occupations not described by these criteria become "professions"?

6. Fully explain how the degree of judgment required in the performance of a particular job can influence the designation of the person performing that job as a "professional" or otherwise.

7. Fully explain how entering into and actively pursuing a professional calling may result in the complete or partial fulfillment of an individual's psychological needs.

8. Select two occupations with which you are familiar, one in health care and one outside of health care, and develop a case both *for* and *against* designating those who pursue this occupation as "professionals."

9. Fully explain why a professional employee is likely to be more loyal to an occupation than to an organization.

10. Describe a health care organization department that includes three or four levels of employees and a mix of professionals and nonprofessionals, and indicate what specific management problems may present themselves given this arrangement of personnel.

QUESTIONS AND ACTIVITIES *(continued)*

11. Explain why a professional employee is likely to be more organizationally mobile than a nonprofessional employee.

12. Explain what is meant by *situational management style,* and provide examples of how it might be applied.

CHAPTER 5

Professional Behavior and Professional Treatment

If you treat an individual as he is, he will stay as he is, but if you treat him as if he were what he ought to be and could be, he will become what he ought to be and could be.
—Johann Wolfgang von Goethe

Almost all absurdity of conduct arises from the imitation of those whom we cannot resemble.
—Samuel Johnson

This Chapter Will:

► Explore the interrelationship between the professional employee's behavior and the organization's treatment of the employee;

► Highlight those aspects of employee behavior for which the manager is most likely to be faced with inconsistencies;

► Review the organization's role—and thus the manager's role—in the treatment of the professional employee.

THE BASIC CONFLICT

The terms *professional behavior* and *professional treatment* represent concepts that should be fairly readily understood. However, although readily *understood*, they are not as readily *defined*. Any attempts at definition usually result in a person recognizing the necessity to consider simultaneously both concepts and their relationship to each other.

Which Came First—?

One ordinarily discovers that professional behavior and professional treatment are highly relative concepts that frequently exist in a chicken-or-egg relationship. Does professional behavior command professional treatment? Does treatment as a professional inspire professional behavior? Or are the two so firmly attached to opposite sides of the same coin that one cannot be touched without affecting the other?

In a practical sense the two concepts are inseparable; professional behavior and professional treatment are indeed opposite sides of the same coin. In

61

many peoples' minds, a given level of professional behavior is associated with professional status, and the organization holds expectations of the employee regarding this level of behavior. Professional employees, both singly and in groups, acquire ideas concerning what constitutes appropriate professional treatment and expect the organization to treat them accordingly. On the other hand, organizations frequently expect so-called professionals to behave in what would be considered a professional manner.

The chicken-or-egg relationship of professional behavior and professional treatment leads to frequent conflict when the expectations of the individual clash with the expectations of the organization. The organizational perspective may suggest that professional treatment is something that the individual earns through professional behavior. However, the individual may hold the opposite perspective and believe that professional behavior is offered in response to professional treatment.

A Two-Way Street

One may argue convincingly—but ultimately incompletely—for either side of the conflict. Much of an individual's treatment as a professional is indeed earned through appropriate behavior; at least continued treatment as a professional is sustained, perhaps rather than earned, through professional behavior. Thorough professional treatment and conscientious professional behavior should ideally exist in full from the beginning of the working relationship. Each should support and sustain the other as the relationship progresses. In brief, behavior and treatment constitute the opposing lanes of an active two-way street on which traffic constantly flows in both directions.

The organization certainly has a responsibility for encouraging continued professional behavior through sustained professional treatment. One springs continually from the other; continued professional treatment is earned through professional behavior, and appropriate professional behavior is acquired by the organization through appropriate treatment.

When the Two Sides Fail to Meet in the Middle

Problems frequently arise when an individual and an organization find it difficult to meet effectively in the middle of a treatment-versus-behavior conflict. For example, the use of time cards required of supposedly professional employees frequently represents an area of conflict. These professionals may be expected to punch time cards, and they may resent doing so because of what they see as the essential inconvenience of the process, or the Big-

Brother-is-watching-you impression they may have of time cards. Or they may simply feel that card punching is clearly the mark of a nonprofessional and contrary to one's professional status. However, card punching, which may well be a holdover requirement of a payroll system approaching the limits of its usefulness, perhaps cannot be eliminated without costly and far-reaching changes.

Unions and Professionals

Professional employees and their organizations are often at extreme odds with each other as to whether collective bargaining is consistent with professional status. The ranks of professionals are often sharply divided as to whether membership in a collective bargaining organization supports or detracts from professionalism. One reason often cited for attempts at union organizing among professional employees is the acquisition of professional treatment for employees. Although unions are frequently able to make sufficient (largely economic) gains for their members, they eventually discover that the factors at the heart of professional treatment, such as respect for the rights and dignity of the individual, are intangibles that cannot be successfully demanded at the bargaining table or mandated by contract. To many who view the organization from the management perspective, the unionized professional has given up some degree of professionalism. However, the view from the employee's side is generally that collective bargaining representation helps to protect professionalism.

The One-to-One Relationship

The relationship between a manager and a professional employee, when it is properly established and working well, often resembles a relationship between peers. Although the supervisor–employee relationship may in fact exist, the surface appearance may be that of a relationship between professional and professional. Most of the time this may be the actual relationship regarding the work of the department, because the manager of the group is usually a professional in the same field as the employee.

With this in mind, we consider professional treatment from the perspectives of both the employee and the organization.

THE EMPLOYEE

There is often a significant difference between being a professional and behaving in a professional manner. It is one thing to possess some degree of professional standing; this is acquired simply by fulfilling the requirements for entry into the profession. Although professional treatment should be provided in full by the organization from the first day of employment, the employee must earn—or in essence pay for—sustained professional treatment through professional behavior. If nothing else, the treatment that one receives is reinforced by one's own behavior.

Status and Standing: Use and Abuse

Entry into a number of professions automatically bestows a certain degree of elevated status upon the individual. Certainly a considerable amount of prestige and status is associated with some of the health professions. Generally inappropriate behavior is evidenced when the employee attempts to trade on this status or prestige for personal reasons, while failing to deliver fully according to the requirements of the position. Among those few professional employees with whom management sometimes experiences problems, it is not unusual to encounter some who expect full professional treatment without delivering professional behavior.

Problems are, of course, likely to develop when an employee appears more than willing to accept the perquisites of the position without behaving accordingly in return. For instance, an individual may take to dodging responsibility or avoiding extra work. The employee may fall into a pattern of working exactly nine to five, regardless of how much or how little work is to be done. The individual may expect—or even demand—extra pay or compensatory time off, but on occasion may nevertheless use the position's supposed exempt status to take time off or otherwise exercise some flexibility. Through such behavior some employees communicate to the organization their desire for the best of both worlds: the salary level and flexibility of the exempt employee, and the extra compensation of the nonexempt employee.

The Lunch-Pail-and-Time-Clock Attitude

Some supposed professionals approach the work situation with a lunch-pail-and-time-clock attitude that is more to be expected of nonexempt employees working in unskilled or semiskilled positions. In some instances this attitude is brought into the organization by the individual; in others it is reinforced, and even encouraged, by the organization (as implicit in the earlier discussion concerning the punching of time cards).

This is not to suggest that the professional employee should be the one who always works more than the basic workday or whose work pattern falls at least partially outside of normally scheduled hours. However, much professional work possesses characteristics that suggest the lunch-pail-and-time-clock attitude may be inappropriate. Many nonprofessional employees perform work that occurs as a series of discrete tasks, many of which may be repetitive. Their work continuity is such that a task may be set aside at quitting time and may be resumed without difficulty at the start of the following day. However, professional work is often of a completely different character—recall the earlier description of professional that referred to intellectual and varied work and the exercise of discretion and judgment—and such work cannot always be set aside at the stroke of 5:00 P.M. and resumed the next morning without loss of continuity.

Control of the Work

The work of the professional is often controlled by the person and not by the clock or by any particular system. For example, the work of the nonexempt tray assembly aide in the food service department is controlled by the speed of the tray line; something must be placed on each tray as it passes by. Likewise the billing clerk in the business office must perform a certain specified task before something else can happen, or before others can do their part. The professional, however, often has a large measure of control over what is to be done, when it is to be done, and how the results are utilized.

The professional's control is much like the manager's control, governed by the individual and rarely if ever by the clock. The professional's work does not always require eight hours' effort beginning and ending at some stroke of the clock. Sometimes longer hours are required; sometimes less time is necessary. However, if a professional employee is consistently working only seven hours, a particular kind of problem exists. If the professional's day is consistently 10 or 11 hours long or longer, this may indicate an entirely different kind of problem. This problem may take one of several forms, or it may simply indicate the presence of an eager, dedicated, and ambitious employee who likes to work. If the behavior reflects the attitude that the employee is simply putting in time, this may be considered as something less than professional. Within reasonable limits, and assuming fair and equitable divisions of work, the professional's focus should be on getting the work done rather that simply putting in a certain amount of time.

Look at *Why* the Person Is Employed

Another perspective from which to view some of these aspects of professional behavior is found in a brief look at the reasons behind the employment of any individual in any capacity. Generally, a nonprofessional employee is employed to do a particular job, and to do so by performing a given set of tasks or by following proscribed procedures. On the other hand, more often than not the professional employee is employed to produce certain results and in doing so has much more flexibility concerning the manner in which those results are achieved. Therefore the professional is engaged to be something of a self-managed worker in a number of respects; thus the emphasis, in the definition of professional, is on the exercise of discretion and judgment.

Behavior of the True Professional

Overall, professional behavior may be seen as behavior that does not seek status as one's primary goal, does not attempt to acquire the advantages of both the exempt and nonexempt employee while avoiding the disadvantages of both, is accepting of the responsibility of the position, is supportive of both the ethics of the profession and the policies of the organization, and is results oriented as opposed to task oriented.

The true professional employee is one who does not abuse the inherent freedom and flexibility of the position in any manner. However, because all employees of professional standing do not always behave as professionals, inappropriate behavior is occasionally encountered. Inappropriate behavior may demand, for instance, relatively close supervision in the accomplishment of tasks that the professional should be expected to handle independently. When a professional employee's behavior seems to necessitate this close supervision, the manager is essentially encountering another circumstance in which the individual is all too willing to accept the rewards of a position without completely fulfilling his or her responsibilities.

Initiative: A Key Concern

Another area related to closeness of supervision in which professional behavior (or lack thereof) is frequently evident is in the exercise of individual initiative. Ideally, all employees at all levels should be encouraged to exercise initiative in certain matters, especially in calling problems or inconsistencies to management's attention. However, true professional behavior suggests that the professional, far more so than the nonprofessional, does not wait to be prodded into action but rather takes positive steps either to deal with problems directly or to call them to the proper persons' attention.

Dedication and the Professional

Relative to dedication, true professional behavior need not be interpreted as requiring one to become a dedicated workaholic. As suggested, those who work long hours and extra days may be doing so because they enjoy what they do. However, with the exception of the occasional push that might be required during an emergency situation or an important major undertaking, the employee need not prove professionalism by constantly working extra hours and extra days. The true workaholic, found primarily among the ranks of managers and professionals, is experiencing some potentially serious problems and is perhaps using the job to compensate for these difficulties. In the long run workaholism, whether arising from an individual's compulsiveness or forced by overly demanding management, is usually harmful to the individual and ultimately damaging to the organization. Far from being the mark of a dedicated professional, workaholism is more often than not an indication of lack of control of one's job. As one author said in putting workaholism into perspective, "Workaholics should be treated, not promoted."[1]

Transference of Expertise

Occasionally a manager may encounter a professional employee who seems to have fallen into the practice of transference of expertise. This tendency surfaces most among persons in the high-skill professions, ones that require considerable intelligence and a significant capacity for study and work. Transference of expertise occurs when the professional is led to automatically assume a level of competence in an area of endeavor other than that of the person's original training. For example, the successful physician who begins to dispense advice on how the organization ought to be run may be exhibiting transference of expertise. This practice finds the professional assuming that he or she is automatically qualified to manage; given that medicine is generally seen as a difficult and important field of learning, some of its practitioners may sometimes see management as a "lesser" field. This behavior reflects the attitude, rarely articulated or even consciously considered by the professional, that "My profession is obviously more difficult than management, and I can handle my profession competently. Because management is a lesser calling than my profession, I am automatically qualified to manage."

There is obviously some measure of sarcasm in the foregoing description of this concept, referred to as transference of expertise. However, the effects can regularly be observed in practice. Although a number of the problems faced by managers in healthcare organizations involve physicians either attempting to tell them how to manage or usurping management prerogatives, the phenomenon of transference of expertise is certainly not limited to physicians. In truth many persons at all organization levels—having in common only the fact of never having been managers—approach management with an attitude that suggests that anyone can do it. Specifically concerning the professional employee, appropriate professional behavior recognizes the difference between advice and interference and further recognizes the manager ultimately responsible for the department.

THE ORGANIZATION

In many relationships with employees, the organization has every right to expect professional behavior. However, in many aspects of employee conduct the behavior exhibited depends largely on the treatment that the organization has extended to the individual.

The Double Standard

The way in which an organization is most likely to err in its treatment of the professional employee is in the creation and perpetuation of a perceived double standard. In other words the organization may treat the individual as a professional at some times and in a contrary fashion at others. This double standard is much like that experienced by many children in the process of growing up. A child, especially an adolescent—close to adulthood in some ways but decidedly still a child in other ways—may be treated as an adult in some respects and as a child in others. "You are certainly old enough to shoulder some responsibility and take care of a few things around here," or so it may go when there is work to be done. However, when a matter of pleasure or privilege arises, the same youngster is likely to hear, "I'm afraid not; you're still too young."

Children detect the double standard the instant they are exposed to it, and so do employees, whether professional or otherwise. Unfortunately, some organizations seem to treat people as professionals only when doing so is convenient for the organization. This inconsistent treatment says to the employee, in effect, "We are really depending on you to do the right thing at the right time and do it in a professional manner—but you had better hit the clock by

8:30 A.M. at the latest and make certain that lunch is only 30 minutes long or you'll be hearing about it."

How the Manager Manages

An extremely important part of professional treatment lies in the manager's leadership style. Authoritarian approaches are far less likely to work with professional employees than with rank-and-file nonprofessionals. On the other hand, consultative and participative approaches—those approaches that stress employee involvement and participation—are far more appropriate to professional employees. Treated long enough as a piece of animated production equipment, a professional eventually either leaves or falls into the habit of behaving as a piece of animated production equipment. In either case the employee's most potentially valuable contributions are lost.

The manager may often find it necessary to differentiate between professionals and nonprofessionals in one-to-one dealings, at least in terms of how one talks with the employee or goes about eliciting appropriate job performance. However, it is essential that all employees, regardless of status, be given equal treatment regarding the organization's policies, benefits, and such, and that all certainly be regarded as equally deserving of equivalent respect. Problems are bound to arise—and it is often the nonprofessionals rather than the professionals who have cause to complain—when one group of employees is treated better than another because of their supposed greater status.

Holding Employees Responsible

All positions in a healthcare organization are important, but professionals usually bear more responsibility than do nonprofessionals. Holding the professional fully responsible for results while subjecting the person to all of the rules applicable to the nonexempt employee is to unfairly limit the freedom and authority of the professional. In any employment relationship, the responsibility for performance and the authority to pursue that performance should coexist in equivalent amounts. However, some organizations limit the professional's ability to perform by failing to provide the degree of freedom and authority essential to facilitate thorough job performance.

Equivalent Treatment

With regard to the policies of the organization, it is appropriate to reward certain classifications of employees with more of some particular benefits.

For instance, many organizations grant more vacation time to managers and professional and technical employees than to most rank-and-file employees. In employee relations matters, however, the professional must be treated exactly the same as the nonprofessional. For instance, it is decidedly unfair—not to mention illegal—to apply a different set of work rules and perhaps a more lenient disciplinary process to a group of employees who are different from others only in that they are professionals. It is true that the professional ordinarily receives a higher salary, and because many employee benefits are tied to pay level the professional is more generously rewarded. This is fine as long as the benefit structure, once established as policy, is applied consistently.

Judgment: Professional Versus Managerial

Frequent conflicts may arise as managers and professionals collide in matters of professional judgment versus managerial judgment. In some such conflicts it is all too common for the authoritarian manager to wield the authority of "the boss" and overrule the professional. In an industry such as health care, in which many judgments involve health and safety, however, the professional has the responsibility for making the judgment call. It falls to both parties to work with each other, on as equal a footing as possible, to resolve such conflicts.

Conflicts of Behavior and Treatment

In general, the organization that expects appropriate behavior from its professional employees may nevertheless discourage such behavior by the treatment that it extends. It is simply wrong for the organization to expect behavior that requires the regular exercise of discretion and judgment, for example, while treating the employee with management's own version of the lunch-pail-and-time-clock attitude. The manager does not generally sit on the shoulders of professional employees; a reasonable degree of operating autonomy—in effect the space in which the discretion and judgment so often referred to may be exercised—is a vital aspect of professional treatment.

Neither should the organization ever take advantage of a professional's status as an exempt employee under the Fair Labor Standards Act. Within this legislation professionals are defined in the same manner as executives and administrators. Some organizations, thankfully a relative few, have been known to hire people in those categories at rates of pay just high enough to avoid payment of overtime and then work them on straight salary for periods consistently in excess of 40 hours per week.

Practices such as that just described represent an organization's attempts to secure for itself the best of both the exempt and nonexempt classifications. Fortunately in most instances in which such practices have been put to the test, the organizations have not prevailed. Usually the jobs of so-called professionals, executives, and administrators involved failed to meet the test of the act in that an unacceptably high percentage of time has been found to be spent on nonexempt work. However, managers in healthcare organizations should be interested to note that the conditions of the Fair Labor Standards Act regarding minimum wages and overtime do not apply to physicians. The long hours that many interns and residents work relative to their compensation are perfectly legal. The final two decades of the twentieth century saw some limitations placed on the number of hours that interns and residents could work in a week, but many can still legally work well in excess of 40 hours per week without running afoul of employment law.

Perhaps elementary to the point of not being worth mentioning, professionals should be provided with job titles that are descriptive of what they do. They should also be provided with appropriate workspace that allows room for professional activities and enhances task accomplishment. In others words one does not engage the services of a certified public accountant and then label that person a bookkeeper, assigned to occupy a two-by-four cubicle beneath a stairway with barely enough room for a small desk.

It is also inappropriate for the organization to expect an employee to be a dedicated workaholic who will be there at all hours. Frequently this kind of pressure is transmitted to the employee from a workaholic manager. Many managers, some consciously but some quite unconsciously, encourage their employees to emulate their own style and behavior. Thus the seemingly dedicated workaholic manager sends signals telling the employees that they are expected to behave in like manner.

It falls to the organization in general and the department manager in particular to set the tone for the relationship with the professional employee. In doing so, the organization and the manager are setting the tone for the response of all professional employees. If an organization's treatment of its professional employees has been consistent and complete in every respect, and yet some individuals have failed to respond with consistently professional behavior, then those cases can be dealt with individually.

NOTE

1. J. M. Fox, *Trapped in the Organization* (Los Angeles: Price/Stern/Sloan Publishers, 1980).

QUESTIONS AND ACTIVITIES

1. Fully explain why it is relatively common in health care to find that some employees who are clearly professionals in terms of their occupations are nevertheless treated in the manner of nonexempt employees, as far as matters of compensation are concerned.

2. Explain why *initiative* and *dedication* would ordinarily be greater concerns for professional employees than for nonprofessional employees.

3. Explain why the relationship between a professional and a department manager will often appear essentially identical to the relationship between peers.

4. Using as many reasons as you are able to provide, explain why in these early years of the twenty-first century you believe unions appear to have targeted groups of health care professionals for organizing.

5. Fully describe two instances in which certain treatment of so-called professionals would appear to be inconsistent with the organization's expectations of these employees.

6. Describe how you believe some supposed professionals take advantage of their professional status, and state how you, as a manager, would address their behavior.

7. Fully explain what you believe is meant by the following sentence from this chapter: *There is often a significant difference between being a professional and behaving in a professional manner.*

8. Describe several forms of employee behavior that you consider inappropriate for professionals and state why these are inappropriate.

9. Put yourself in the position of a health care professional seeking employment. List five or six conditions, policies, or practices you would like to find in whatever organization you go to work for, and explain why the presence or absence of these could affect your choice of organization.

10. Explain why some nonmanaging professionals seem to automatically assume the ability to manage. What does this say about their view of management versus their view of any individual profession?

11. Fully explain why the requirement to use time cards or time sheets is frequently resisted by some professional employees as being unprofessional.

12. You first are to offer an *opinion* as to whether union membership is or is not consistent with professionalism, and second, provide as many reasons as you can think of to justify your opinion.

CHAPTER 6

Professional Mobility: Up, Across, or Out?

What we see depends mainly on what we look for.
—John Lubbock

This Chapter Will:

► Examine the professional employee's limited ability to move horizontally within the health care organization;

► Introduce the concept of career ladders in relation to the professional's growth potential, and identify the opportunities for and the barriers to vertical movement;

► Explore the dimension of employment mobility in which the professional has the strongest advantage: the ability to move from organization to organization essentially as a "free agent."

ACROSS AND UP: INTERNAL MOBILITY

Horizontal Mobility

Nonprofessionals Have the Edge in Horizontal Movement

Without additional training, the professional employee generally has somewhat limited horizontal mobility within the organization. On the other hand, the nonprofessional employee is quite often horizontally mobile within the organization. The housekeeping worker can conceivably transfer to food service and become a kitchen worker; the kitchen worker can transfer to a housekeeping job; the clerk in the business office can fill a clerk's position in the human resources department or elsewhere. Many nonprofessionals hold jobs that are considered entry-level positions, and because employees are usually oriented to such positions via on-the-job training, it matters not whether an employee comes from outside the organization or from another department within the same organization. Internal transfers are often to the advantage of the organization because an employee coming from one department into another will already be familiar with the organization and many of its practices.

Obstacles to Professionals' Horizontal Movement

The professional or technical employee, however, is a specialist of sorts and thus cannot readily move from department to department. Some moves can be made, but these depend on the presence of the appropriate qualifications. For example, a large hospital's nursing department, emergency department, mental health center, ambulatory services division, and many smaller departments may use registered nurses. Although a nurse may have several places to go, many other specialists have no other place to go. It is doubtful, for instance, that a physical therapist can readily go to work in any department other than physical therapy, or that a medical laboratory technologist can go anywhere other than another section of the laboratory department (perhaps by moving from chemistry to hematology, for example).

For most professional and technical employees, a move to another department within the same organization entails a move to another occupational career ladder, and this requires qualification in another specialty. Such diversification may sometimes be accomplished by obtaining additional training that builds on one's existing background. A radiological technician might acquire additional knowledge and credentials as a nuclear medicine technician, or the registered nurse can take a shorter route to becoming a physician's assistant because of his or her nursing background. However, many health occupations are so different from each other that a move from one to another is impractical without extensive retraining It is difficult to conceive of a social worker becoming a medical technologist without starting from scratch in laboratory work (except perhaps for a few fundamentals that might be acquired in either kind of educational program).

A Variety of Specialties

Consider the diversity of technical and professional specialties found in a modern health care organization, especially a full-service acute-care hospital. Activities include nursing, radiology, laboratory, respiratory therapy, social work, biomedical engineering, occupational therapy, accounting, and therapeutic dietetics, among others. In most instances, at any level above entry it is possible to change from one specialty to another only by adopting a second career; that is, by becoming trained and credentialed in another specialty. Going from one profession to another may take slightly less time and effort for a professional trained in one field than for a completely untrained worker. For example, a degreed biomedical engineer and a graduate accountant may have a few undergraduate courses in common (e.g., English and economics) so that the route to a career change is shorter than for someone with no degree at all. Nevertheless, the biomedical engineer who wants to change to accounting would have to make up perhaps two or more years of academic study to qualify minimally as an accountant.

Specialization and Horizontal Mobility

The more narrowly defined and specialized an occupation becomes, the more difficult it becomes to move into or out of that occupation within the work organization. There is more than a grain of truth in the description of a *specialist* as someone who strives to learn more and more about less and less. As one further specializes, one's knowledge grows in depth but it applies to an increasingly narrower range in scope. There is a strong tendency toward specialization in health care. This tendency, developing in response to rapidly expanding medical technology, has prompted many specialized occupations to spring up on their own or to splinter off from other occupations. Technological progress in medicine has brought specialization into health care, and specialization makes it increasingly more difficult for the health care professional to move horizontally within an organization.

Horizontal mobility in the health care organization is severely limited for the professional or technical employee, regardless of the size of the organization. However, such is not the case regarding vertical mobility—the opportunity to move upward in the organization's hierarchy. Vertical mobility may exist to a considerable extent, to a modest or limited extent, or not at all depending on the size of the institution and the institution's use of a particular specialty.

Vertical Mobility: Career Ladders

Moving Up Rather than Across

Career ladders are a popular concept in health care organizations. A *career ladder* is simply the series of internal advancements available to an employee who remains within a particular occupational field. For most professional and technical employees, the career ladders existing in health care organizations are strictly separated from each other by education, credentials, and experience. Certainly the specialized education, the requirements for degrees and diplomas in special fields, and the necessary credentials have served to clearly separate most specialties from each other, define entry levels, and prevent horizontal movement among occupations.

Most of the professional's mobility within an organization is vertical, and essentially all of this mobility is restricted to the individual's specific career ladder. Room for vertical movement depends largely on the size of the organization: there may be a number of levels on a career ladder in a medium to large institution, but perhaps only one level at a small institution. For example, in a particular hospital in the 400- to 500-bed range, there are four levels on the physical therapy career ladder and five levels on the respiratory therapy career ladder. In another hospital in the same region, a rural institution of fewer than 60 beds, physical therapy and respiratory therapy have one level each to their career ladders, as these functions are one-person departments.

Because it is nearly impossible to move from one professional career ladder to another, the most possible movement is vertical. However, climbing one's own career ladder is not necessarily as easy as a career-ladder chart might make it appear to be.

Climbing the Ladder: The Biomedical Engineering Example

Table 6–1 is a career ladder that shows the positions in the biomedical engineering department of a hospital in the 600- to 700-bed range. At first glance it appears as though the steps in the biomedical engineering career ladder offer sufficient room for movement to satisfy even an ambitious employee's need for growth opportunity. However, it is necessary to examine the hierarchy of positions in light of what is required of the employee to make each upward move.

A person who enters this career ladder at the bottom—as a biomedical technician I with only two to four years of appropriate experience—would probably have to acquire an associate's degree before moving to biomedical technician II. This would require the equivalent of up to two years of academic work. To move to junior biomedical engineer would require a bachelor's degree, another two years of full-

---

Table 6–1   Career Ladder for Biomedical Engineering

Position	Requirements
Department manager	Master's degree in biomedical electrical, or electronics engineering, plus five or more years of appropriate experience.
Senior biomedical engineer	Bachelor's degree in biomedical, electrical, or electronics engineering, plus three to five years of appropriate experience.
Junior biomedical engineer	Bachelor's degree in biomedical, electrical, or electronics engineering, plus two to four years of appropriate experience.
Biomedical technician II	Associate's degree in electronics technology, plus one to two years of appropriate experience.
Biomedical technician I	Associate's degree in electronics technology or two to four years of appropriate experience.

time college work (or several more years of part-time college work), not to mention the added experience that must be accumulated. The move to senior biomedical engineer may be relatively easy to make on experience alone, assuming that an opening is made available, but an eventual move to manager of biomedical engineering requires a master's degree, entailing another two years or more of academic work.

Overall, the individual who begins at the bottom of the ladder on experience alone must acquire up to six years of college education to move all the way up to the top position in the department. Also to be reckoned with are the years of experience to be acquired along the way, and the sometimes lengthy wait for higher positions to open up. The five-step career ladder for biomedical engineering may be a reality, but as the illustration suggests, it is necessary for the employee to take the initiative to reach outside of the organization for education that may be costly, difficult, and time-consuming.

Regardless of the difficulty of pursuing career growth within the biomedical engineering department, the employees on this career ladder are at least able to see the possibility for growth. In many organizations, though, this is not the case. For instance, a much smaller hospital may have only one person in the biomedical engineering function. In this case, biomedical engineering would be a classic dead-end function: the incumbent tops out in the entry step because it is the only step. As a true specialist, the individual has essentially no opportunity for horizontal movement to another career ladder, and no more than an extremely slim chance to rise into administration.

The Longest Climb: The Nursing Example

In most health care organizations, the lengthiest professional career ladder is in nursing service. Consider the nursing department career ladder (Table 6–2) adapted from the same institution that provided the biomedical engineering illustration.

Once again, a multilevel hierarchy suggests that there is more than adequate room within nursing for advancement. However, the same barriers are present: a nursing assistant cannot advance at all within nursing without acquiring education and credentials; an L.P.N. can likewise make no move without acquiring more education and additional credentials; a registered nurse with only an associate's degree or diploma can make just one move, to the position of team leader, without having to acquire a bachelor's degree; and the bachelor's degreed head nurse can conceivably move up only as far as nursing

Table 6–2   Career Ladder in Nursing

Position	Requirements
Director of nursing	Master's degree, R.N., plus ten years of management experience.
Assistant director	Master's degree, R.N., plus five to ten years of management experience.
Nursing supervisor	Bachelor's degree, R.N. (master's preferred), plus five years of nursing experience.
Staff development instructor	Bachelor's degree, R.N. (master's preferred), plus five years of nursing experience or two years of nursing education experience.
Head nurse/unit manager	Bachelor's degree, R.N., plus three years of nursing experience.
Team leader	R.N. (bachelor's degree, diploma, or associate's degree), plus two years of nursing experience.
Staff nurse	R.N. (bachelor's degree, diploma, or associate's degree).
Staff L.P.N.	Licensed practical nurse.
Nursing assistant	High school graduate or equivalent.

supervisor before the absence of a master's degree becomes a barrier to advancement.

The opportunity for advancement within nursing is clearly there, but the path is neither easily nor readily negotiated. It is necessary for the individual to reach out and independently pursue the qualifications required for advancement, thus devoting considerable time and effort to the task while remaining active on a job (or periodically dropping out of the workforce to pursue additional studies). The work organization is generally supportive of such growth and often provides tuition aid, but the responsibility for this growth—and certainly the work that is involved—falls to the individual.

It seems to matter little that the chances of making the journey all the way to the top are relatively slim, even for one with all of the prerequisite qualifications and necessary credentials. After all, the organization portrayed in the foregoing example may have 700 to 800 or more registered nurses. Only one registered nurse can be the director of nursing, and chances are at least fifty-fifty that a new director, when one is needed, will come from outside the organization. The career ladder need not be easy to climb; usually it is not. Rather, what is important is that the career ladder exists. As long as advancement is possible, no matter how difficult, it still has a positive effect. Although some people are overwhelmed by the career ladder to the extent that they never attempt to climb it, many nevertheless recognize that the opportunity, no mater how slim, is there and that advancement is possible.

Topping Out

It should be clear to any growth-oriented professional employee that advancement possibilities are limited by the number of levels on the career ladder and the number of positions available at each level. Within any particular organization, one can go only as far as the structure permits.

Organizational limitations can cause problems in varying degrees as employees move toward the top of a career ladder. Employees tend more and more to become caught between drives to satisfy various needs; for example, the need for job security versus the need for advancement and achievement.

A particular problem is sometimes presented by the nonmanagerial specialist who tops out; that is, who reaches the highest nonmanagerial position on the function's career ladder. (In the case of the biomedical engineering career ladder, this would be someone who attains the position of senior biomedical engineer.) The person who tops out and remains there for some time (the length of time varies, depending on the person) may begin to feel the effects of limited opportunity. Additionally, feelings of a lack of expanding challenge, or a lessening of interest in the work, may develop. After time, these noticeable limitations may be joined by the knowledge that one has reached the maximum salary grade for the job, and that no more money can be forthcoming except as the grade structure may happen to advance periodically.

When an employee tops out in a position, he or she often begins to experience a reordering of motivating forces as structural limitations are recognized and felt. As a professional or nonprofessional, the employee who has reached the top of the pay scale in the career ladder's top nonmanagerial job can present some difficult, long-term motivational problems. (See Chapter 7, especially the section concerning the dead-end employee.)

Into Management

The top rung of a function's career ladder is the position of department manager. In most organizations, and especially in health care organizations, it is rare that a department head managing a specialized activity is not trained as a specialist in that activity. The manager of biomedical engineering is usually a biomedical engineer; the director of nursing service is ordinarily a registered nurse; the chief of occupational therapy is invariably an occupational therapist.

Although the department head position is usually the target position for persons climbing the career ladder, all such persons are not necessarily suited to management. It is true that the good specialist—the one who knows the occupation well and performs well—is more likely than the mediocre performer to be promoted into management. This is as it should be; one can hardly imagine why higher management would ever consciously promote a poor performer. However, the fact that one is a good specialist is no guarantee that the person will become a good manager. Nevertheless, work organizations continue to promote outstanding workers into departmental management only to see many of them become poor or marginally effective managers. This will continue in most organizations, essentially because there is no way to continue rewarding the outstanding performer who has reached the top of the grade other than promoting that person into management. The only exception is the occasional organization's success at implementing "parallel path progression," as discussed in the following section. (For a discussion of the problems of the specialist-manager, refer to Chapter 10.)

The department head—the professional at the top of the career ladder—may aspire to administration. Such a move is possible, but chances are so slim that for all practical purposes the possibility is often merely theoretical. Administrative positions increasingly are being filled by persons who are trained as professional administrators, severely limiting the opportunities for administrators to come up through the ranks. Also, such a move makes it necessarily for the professional to virtually abandon the specialty, at least as far as active practice and involvement are concerned, and take on the full-time role of a management generalist.

Parallel Path Progression

As noted above, parallel path progression presents a method of continuing to substantively recognize continued good performance by some certain valuable employees without promoting them into management. Some organizations have established parallel growth paths such that more senior and more accomplished employees can acquire pay and benefits equivalent to those associated with some management positions. This is done by creating two, three, or more senior levels and extending the technical or professional scale upward such that it significantly overlaps the management scale. In the most effective parallel path progression systems, advancement to the senior levels comes about through a combination of performance on the job and fulfillment of certain optional educational requirements over and above the basic requirements of the occupation. In many such systems employees must pass an examination to move up a level, and it is not unusual for there to be a time-in-grade requirement; that is, a requirement that one must function at a particular level for a certain minimum period of time (perhaps one year) before attempting to attain the next level.

Even in the presence of parallel path progression, employees can still top out at their pay scales. However, by having to progress through perhaps three or four levels it will take an individual several years longer to top out than it would were there no such system in place. Parallel path progression is highly appropriate for technical and professional employees who wish to continue working and advancing in their chosen fields without pursuing movement into management.

Other Directions

Restricted internal mobility may present large problems or it may present no problem at all; it depends entirely on the needs and drives of the individual professional. To those persons for whom continuing advancement is a pressing need, the organization eventually presents limitations. As persons move up their respective career ladders toward the top of the organizational pyramid, they begin to encounter shortages of positions. Higher up on the ladder there are fewer jobs, and these fewer jobs may not turn over with any great frequency.

When growth-oriented professionals look up the ladder and see no positions available, they begin to look toward other organizations. In those other organizations, positions may open sooner because people with appropriate qualifications are not available internally (e.g., an organization may need another biomedical engineer but there is no degreed candidate in house). The temptation to move to another organization is felt by those to whom advancement is important.

Professional and technical employees are severely limited horizontally and somewhat limited vertically within the organization. However, regarding external mobility—the ability to move to other organizations—professionals fare better than most other employees.

OUT: INTERORGANIZATIONAL MOBILITY

Specialization and Interorganizational Movement

As compared with nonprofessionals, professional employees generally enjoy greater ability to move from organization to organization. In considering all kinds of work that may be done in a health care organization, interorganizational mobility generally increases as a worker moves up the ladder of specialization. That is, the less specialized employee is generally less mobile than the more specialized employee.

The nonprofessional employee who comes to work in the organization must ordinarily learn, in addition to the policies and practices of the organization, how to do the work itself. More often than not this business of learning is accomplished through on-the-job training. The message that the organization is conveying to the nonprofessional at the time of hire is "We have work that we want you to do, and we will show you how to do it." During times of a normal job market, the nonprofessional—particularly the unskilled or semi-skilled worker—finds it more difficult to change organizations than does the professional. As the job market gets tighter, the nonprofessional's ability to change organizations becomes even more limited.

The professional, however, receives a different message from the organization at the time of hire: "We are hiring you to do your kind of work. We simply want you to do it in our particular environment, and do it in a manner consistent with our organizational objectives." The professional is educated in at least the fundamentals of an occupational specialty. This implies certain minimum qualifications, and the specific position requires these minimum qualifications. The professional may receive some on-the-job training to provide orientation to specific tasks, and certainly is made knowledgeable of the organization's policies and practices. However, the organization considers the newly hired professional as at least minimally qualified to perform a certain kind of work before starting. As compared with the nonprofessional, the professional is less limited by general economic conditions but is more likely to be limited by the market for a particular profession. As long as one's profession is not overcrowded, the professional finds it much easier to change organizations.

Moving Easiest: The High-Skill Professional

In general, the high-skill professional can move the easiest as long as the particular occupation is not in a state of oversupply. Mobility is often limited by oversupply, an overcrowding that can be either temporary or long lasting and either regional or widespread. The professional, and especially the high-skill professional, may remain considerably mobile even when a given region is experiencing oversupply. It is not uncommon for a professional to be recruited from afar and, depending on one's degree of specialization and extent of importance to the recruiting organization, be paid some if not all of his or her interview and moving expenses. Rarely, if ever, does a nonprofessional in health care receive a moving allowance.

Factors Influencing Mobility

To a considerable extent, mobility is influenced by the urgency of the organization's needs and the market conditions relative to the supply of persons in a given specialty. Within specific groups of professionals, however, mobility is most often influenced by a number of personally related factors that include

- an individual's economic needs;
- an individual's other needs (e.g., challenge, accomplishment, or social or family group affiliations);
- geographic preferences; and
- gender and marital status.

For example, at times regional shortages of nurses have resulted in the availability of many seemingly attractive positions for registered nurses. In many areas the needs have been sufficiently acute to give rise to the use of generous moving allowances, inflated salaries, and other benefits to induce nurses to relocate. However, some recruiters offering generous packages find that they are appealing to only a limited segment of the total population of nurses. Some 96 percent of nurses are female. Many female nurses are unmarried, but the majority of female nurses are married and many of them are not the primary wage earners in their families. The mobility of these nurses is limited; they do not ordinarily consider themselves available for long-distance moves—*long distance* being a move that takes one more than a reasonable commuting distance from home, with the precise meaning of *reasonable* being another factor that varies from person to person.

A nurse's employment frequently hinges on a spouse's employment. The opportunity for nurse employment may stand as one of many factors in a family relocation decision, but ordinarily it is not the determining factor.

So-called long-distance moves aside, matters of economics and commuting distance present some varying barriers to mobility even within geographic areas of fairly limited size. Once again registered nurses provide some pertinent illustrations. Even in times of a relative shortage of nurses, hospitals in some metropolitan centers have managed to keep the level of nursing vacancies under control. However, smaller hospitals in outlying areas may remain critically short of nurses. Most nurses are concentrated in metropolitan areas; when they can find work relatively close to home, most do so instead of opting for a lengthy commute to an institution at which the pay is probably less than it would be near home. Even when there have been more job-seeking nurses than available positions—a condition experienced less and less frequently during this first decade of the twenty-first century—many nurses opt to wait for an opening in a metropolitan hospital rather than deciding to travel an hour or more to and from an outlying institution. Looking at the composition of nursing staffs of small hospitals in rural areas, one often discovers that those areas are home for many of the nurses who work there because of family ties and perhaps spousal employment.

Regardless of differences among various groups of professionals, however, professionals as a class enjoy a greater degree of interorganizational mobility than nonprofessionals. At almost all times, even during periods of recession and economic retrenchment, a certain amount of mobility exists among health professionals because of both normal turnover and chronic shortages in some specialties.

The "Free-Agent" Mentality

When drawing a parallel between the health care professions and the world of the professional athlete, we recognize some similarities between the professional athlete and the working health care professional. Most people are familiar with the concept of free agency in professional sports. After playing for a particular length of time and developing (one would hope) a marketable level of expertise, an athlete is able to sell as a free agent his or her future services to whatever team offers the most attractive deal. It is the sport or the game that holds the player's primary loyalty. Loyalty to a specific team is transitory, often lasting only until the end of a contractual term, at which time the "loyalty" may be transferred to another team. In this fashion an athlete may play for several teams over the course of a career.

As mentioned earlier, the professional employee's loyalty often tends toward occupation over organization, while the nonprofessional is likely to feel stronger ties to organization rather than occupation. The professional often has experienced divided loyalty while the nonprofessional has not. The presence of the free-agent mentality, increasingly evident among health care professionals, suggests that divided loyalty has given way to a preponderance of loyalty to profession—and thus loyalty to self. We therefore find that a significant percentage of health care professionals are constantly alert to the opportunity to move to another "team" if the inducements are sufficiently attractive.

Health care organizations are susceptible to the movement of free-agent employees at all times, and are especially so during times of staff shortages, when organizations compete for scarce professionals by offering various inducements in the effort to attract needed skills. One cannot readily predict what will induce any particular professional to change organizations. For example, all other factors—pay, benefits, professional environment, and such —being equal from one organization to another, a given professional might change organizations for a reason as simple as working closer to home. Another professional, interested in continuing education and development, might move because of an attractive tuition assistance program. A different one might move for more money, a more attractive benefits package, or what might be perceived as a more attractive working environment. Yet another might be swayed to move for what is often the strongest lure to the free-agent professional, the person solidly dedicated to profession over organization: A more challenging professional situation that allows greater freedom and increased responsibility.

The free agent will likely be a strong factor in the interorganizational movement of health care personnel for the coming decade or two. The only condition capable of stifling free agency altogether would be a considerable oversupply in all affected occupations, something unlikely to occur in the foreseeable future.

Mobility Is a Matter of Degree

An occupation's degree of interorganizational mobility is directly related to the ability of a given number of persons to do that kind of work. Because almost anyone can be trained in a reasonable time to do many kinds of nonprofessional work, these workers can come from a variety of sources. (There are limits to this claim. For instance, not everyone can be trained quickly to do certain kinds of office work. However, persons with office skills exist in such relative abundance that such positions rarely remain open for long.) On the other hand professional work is such that only a finite number of qualified people can do it, and many of these qualified people may already be employed by other organizations.

In addition, the nonprofessional who wishes to change organizations has only experience to sell while the professional has both experience and credentials to sell. The professional's credentials—degree, license, certification, and such—are, if not an absolute guarantee of a position, at least a ticket that opens the door of the employment office. In effect this ticket says, "Here is a person who can (or is supposed to be able to) do this particular kind of work." Given the health care industry's tendency to rely heavily on credentialing, certain health care professionals may find that they encounter frequent efforts to entice them to other organizations, especially when their skills are in relatively short supply. In this respect, professionals being lured elsewhere by the prospect of more favorable employment are fully mobile, while nonprofessionals are completely immobile.

In summary, it is safe to conclude that when interorganizational mobility is at its best, it is best for everyone, professional and nonprofessional. When interorganizational mobility is at its worst, it is at its worst for everyone. In either case, however, and regardless of the state of employment opportunities at any given time, interorganizational mobility is always better for the professional than for the nonprofessional.

QUESTIONS AND ACTIVITIES

1. Fully explain how a period of recession is likely to affect mobility for both professional and nonprofessional employees.

2. Is it important for all employees to be able to see the existence of the opportunity for growth and advancement? How could the existence of this opportunity be important to employees who never take advantage of it?

3. Explain in detail why horizontal mobility is severely limited for professional employees in most health care organizations.

4. Describe the results likely to occur when all department management positions are filled from outside of the organization. Also, describe the possible results of filling all such positions from within the organization.

5. Describe in detail the ways in which a system of *parallel path progression* differs from an occupational *career ladder.*

6. Using a specific occupational example, explain how a particular professional employee might make a move to another career ladder.

7. Select an occupational specialty likely to be found in a large health care organization and develop a theoretical career ladder for that specialty, including designation of what is required to move upward through each level.

QUESTIONS AND ACTIVITIES *(continued)*

8. The manager of a department is expected to be well versed in both the department's specialty and in management. Which area of knowledge, if either, is more important to the manager, and why?

9. It is acknowledged that it is often advantageous to fill open positions via internal transfer, as existing employees know the organization's policies, procedures, and the like. What, if any, might be the disadvantages of filling positions in this manner?

10. Identify one health care occupation that is known to—or at least appears to—have evolved, or "split off," from another occupation. Describe its apparent evolution and outline a possible career ladder for it.

11. Occasionally the health care organizations in a given geographic area will become competitive in bidding for the services of a limited group of professionals. Describe both the advantages and disadvantages of this process.

12. Some organizations' hiring criteria allow for flexible combinations of education and experience. For example, the hiring criteria might require a master's degree and two years experience or a bachelor's degree and six years experience. Take a position either for or against such flexible criteria and fully explain your position.

CHAPTER 7

Motivation and the Professional

It is far easier to perceive and to criticize the aspects
in motivation theory than to remedy them.
Abraham H. Maslow

This Chapter Will:

► Review some of the significant features of the more widely known theories of employee motivation.

► Examine the significance of work itself as the primary source of employee motivation.

► Explore the extent of the manager's influence on the factors that seem to motivate people to work.

► Examine commonly accepted motivational factors specifically as they may apply to professional employees.

► Look briefly at turnover among professional employees and consider the special case of the dead-end employee.

ABUNDANCE OF MOTIVATION THEORIES

A Theory Is Only a Theory

The opening quotation, from the frequently cited writings of Abraham H. Maslow, suggests that all well-known theoretical approaches to human motivation possess identifiable weaknesses and shortcomings. It is indeed true that the theories carry a tone of universality about them; all of the theories that deal in any way with the motivation to work suggest that if management puts interest, challenge, and opportunity for accomplishment into a job, then the worker will perform as desired. As agreeable to reason as this contention may appear, though, it does not always work.

All popular motivation theories are logically formulated, and all are agreeable to reason. They make sense. At times the theories make so much sense that when they fail to work as anticipated, management's first reaction is to question the manner in which the theories were applied. When managers' behavior in applying the theories cannot be found at fault, then perhaps the theories themselves are questioned. A theory, after all, is only a theory. A rule or principle, or whatever we care to call it, enjoys the force or status of *law* only if it is proven to apply in all possible instances, and by definition a theory has not been proven in all instances. As concerns apparently unsuccessful applications of motivation theory, seldom does management go further to consider whether they should question the behavior of the people to whom the theories are applied.

The basic motivation to work is often found to vary from person to person, and much of the time it varies significantly. As a result, the popular theories of motivation work well with some people but not at all with other people. The motivation to work is simply not present to an equivalent degree in all persons. The importance of work as part of one's life varies from top priority to last place. For a considerable number of people work is, and forever will be, no more than a means to a number of ends.

People are different from each other. Work can be "just a job" or it can encompass the pursuit of a career or even a calling. It can be the means to fulfillment in all other areas of life, or it can be a major area of fulfillment itself.

Maslow in Brief

Probably the best-known motivation theory is that advanced in 1943 by Abraham Maslow.[1] In his widely studied work, Maslow argued that people, in their drive to advance themselves and improve the quality of their lives, tended to move upward through a hierarchy of needs. According to this theory, a person who achieves satisfaction of needs at a given level then tends to seek satisfaction of needs at the next highest level in the hierarchy. Maslow's need hierarchy proceeds from lowest to highest level through the following progression:

- *Physiological needs*—the most fundamental needs, such as the need for food to eat and air to breathe; the things required to sustain life at an elementary level.

- *Safety needs*—the need to be protected from the elements, and from harm from others, and the need to be free of the fear of deprivation of the means to sustain life.

- *Love needs*—the need to be accepted by others, to be accepted into group membership, and to be included in activities and affairs that involve others.

- *Esteem needs*—the need to achieve, to acquire status and recognition, and to gain the respect of others.

- *The need for self-actualization*—the need to pursue one's own ideal, to rise above all other concerns, and attain that which provides the most personal fulfillment to the individual.

In Search of Satisfaction

In terms relevant to the world of work, a person works toward the satisfaction of physiological needs by obtaining employment and thus generating an income with which to acquire the necessities of life. The person proceeds to acquire shelter and whatever other protection may be desired, and also seeks reasonable assurance that the income stream will not be disrupted. Whereas initially the person may have been interested only in getting a job and securing the necessities of life, once gainfully employed his or her attention turns to remaining employed. The desire for job security is a common sign of a perceived safety need.

With a steady income acquired and a reasonable sense of job security, attention is likely to turn toward the love needs, and the person seeks acceptance into various work or social groups. Later the esteem needs arise, and the person desires recognition for work done or for other accomplishments. Ultimately the person proceeding through the entire need hierarchy may strive to realize a highly personal "dream." Such is the case with many who drop out of supposedly conventional involvements or abandon apparently successfully or lucrative careers to go their own way—like the master toolmaker who abandons a well-paid position in his middle years to become a schoolteacher at a much lower salary, the wealthy farmer who sells his immense holdings to become an unpaid agricultural advisor in an undeveloped country, and the corporate executive who leaves the boardroom to open a restaurant, because that was what he had always wanted to do. (Some persons of course realize their dreams without necessarily dropping out, but rather by achieving a measure of financial security on retirement from one line of work before stepping out in personal directions.)

A Simpler Hierarchy

Other motivational theorists have advanced a simpler hierarchy comprising three levels:

1. Physiological needs, that combine Maslow's first two levels (physiological and safety needs) into a single level concerned with sustenance and protection.

2. Sociological needs, directly equivalent to Maslow's love needs, or the need for a sense of belonging.

3. Psychological needs, that combine Maslow's esteem needs and the need for self-actualization.

This three-level hierarchy represents a convenient way of viewing human needs: first, the concerns for the body; second, the concerns for relations with others; and finally, the concerns for one's soul and intellect.

The principal problem in relating these theories of human motivation to the world of work lies in the fact that many people simply never expect fulfillment of higher-order needs—primarily the psychological needs—from work. To many, work is simply a necessary evil and one does the minimum amount possible for the maximum reward that can be attained. Some people work only as a means for acquiring food, shelter, and the resources with which to pursue other interests.

The Herzberg Perspective

The Maslow theory alone cannot supply all of the answers that a manager needs, but it is invaluable as a starting point and is especially helpful when considered along with other approaches. Another approach of considerable value is the motivation-hygiene theory of Frederick Herzberg.[2]

Although Herzberg postulated a needs hierarchy similar to that of Maslow, he focused instead on relating motivation and need satisfaction to work and closely examined factors comprising the job and surrounding the job. He concluded that true motivators are inherent in the work and that what he called hygiene factors—those things making up the environment surrounding the work—are not motivators but rather are potential dissatisfiers. Herzberg's work suggests that managers must focus on jobs and their content as central to the motivation to work, and look at salaries, benefits, working conditions, and such as factors in the environment that must be reinforced periodically to stave off dissatisfaction.

With this in mind, we can proceed to examine the factors related to an individual's employment with a view toward determining which factors may be true motivators and which may be primarily environmental.

MOTIVATION IN THE WORKING RELATIONSHIP

Motivating Factors Versus Environmental Factors

The factors having a bearing on people's relationship with their work can be divided into two groups: *motivating factors* and *environmental factors*. Motivating factors can and do truly motivate a person to perform. Environmental factors, though not functioning directly as motivators, do, for better or worse, influence employee satisfaction.

The True Motivators

The true motivating factors are, as Herzberg suggests, inherent in the work. The key word that can be used to describe these motivating factors is *opportunity*. The sources of motivation are the opportunity to

- learn (to acquire new knowledge)
- achieve
- perform work that is interesting and challenging
- do meaningful work
- assume responsibility
- become involved in determining how the work is done.

Environmental Factors: Potential Dissatisfiers

Environmental factors, on the other hand, exist in all aspects of the employee's relationship to the organization and the employment situation. Even if the environmental factors are acceptable, they do not necessarily motivate. However, if they are *not* acceptable, they can lead directly to employee dissatisfaction. Environmental factors can be arranged into five categories:

1. *Communication*

   - Appreciation of one's efforts; praise when it is due
   - Knowledge of the organization's activities and intentions; inclusion in the employer's goals and plans
   - Knowledge of where one stands within the organization at any given time; appraisal
   - Confidentiality in personal dealings with management; tactful disciplining and reasonable privacy.

2. *Growth Potential*

   - The opportunity for advancement; career ladders and promotional paths
   - Encouragement in growth and advancement; skill training, tuition assistance for formal education, and management training for potential supervisors.

3. *Personnel Policies*

- Reasonable accommodation of personal needs, as in work scheduling, vacation scheduling, sick time benefits, and so forth
- Reasonable feeling of job security
- Organizational loyalty to employees
- Respect for an individual's origins, background, and beliefs
- Fair and consistent treatment relative to that afforded other employees.

4. *Salary Administration*

- Fair salary and benefits relative to others in the organization, in the community, and in one's specific occupation

5. *Working Conditions*

- The physical working conditions relative to what is expected or desired.

THE MANAGER'S ROLE

The department manager can influence both motivating factors and environmental factors. However, the extent of possible influence depends partly on the job (specifically, what the manager has to work with) and partly on the organization, and in particular, how much latitude the individual manager is allowed.

For all employees, the manager has at least some ability to arouse motivation and to prevent dissatisfaction from taking over. As far as true motivating factors are concerned, the nature of professional work suggests that the manager has considerable opportunity to stimulate motivation. Certainly the manager has more such opportunity with the professional employee that with the nonprofessional employee.

The true motivating factors—the opportunities listed previously—represent that capacity for the fulfillment of needs that are largely, if not entirely, psychological. As compared with the nonprofessional, the professional employee is more likely to be operating on a level of psychological need fulfillment. This should suggest to the manager that the professional employee would be more effectively managed through an open, participative management style that allows the employee the maximum possible opportunity for self-determination.

Let us now consider the manager's likely impact on the five categories of environmental factors surrounding the professional's work.

The Manager and the Environmental Factors

1. **Communication.** The immediate manager is always the key to communication with employees at all levels. Whether professional or nonprofessional, an employee's overall level of satisfaction often hinges completely, or at least in large part, on communication that is controlled by the manager. Communication serves many important needs in answering for the employee many questions such as, How am I doing? Am I appreciated? Am I trusted and regarded with respect? Am I kept advised of what is happening in the organization? Am I treated as truly a part of the organization? These questions and more are answered both directly and indirectly by the manager in the all-important one-to-one relationship with the employee.

2. **Growth potential.** The manager has somewhat limited influence in the area of growth potential. Quite simply, the manager cannot create opportunities that may not be there because there are few openings for promotions or because short, restrictive career ladders are involved. The manager can, however, adopt a positive attitude that encourages employees to fix their sights on existing opportunities (limited though they may be, their existence suggests that someone will advance now and then).

3. **Personnel policies.** As a member of the larger management group, the individual manager may have input into the formulation of personnel policies. The extent of possible input varies from organization to organization, depending on top management's philosophy of policy making. Regardless of the extent of one's involvement in setting policy, however, the manager always has a key role in assuring the consistent application of personnel policies to all employees. Because inconsistency of treatment tends to be a major dissatisfier for many employees, this places considerable responsibility in the hands of the manager.

4. **Salary administration.** Ordinarily, the manager has little or no role in determining the salary structure of the organization. However, in hiring and promoting people and in rating pay raises, the manager may well have a key role in the consistent and equitable application of the salary structure. Often the principal determinant of an employee's level of satisfaction with salary is that person's perception of how well he or she is paid relative to others, especially others of comparable skill who do the same kind of work.

5. **Working conditions.** The manager has an active role in watching out for the well-being of employees. Something as seemingly simple as inadequate lighting in the office or insufficient space in the parking lot can lead to dissatisfaction if not acted on. The manager, in many ways the advocate of the employee, in part ensures that the job gets done by making certain that working conditions are reasonable or at least tolerable. The manager should serve as a willing channel through which complaints about working conditions are aired and problems are reported and corrected.

THE PROFESSIONAL'S MOTIVATORS

As alluded to in Chapter 4, the professional, as compared with the nonprofessional, is more likely to

- aspire to growth within the occupation and organization and aspire to earn increasingly larger amounts of money;
- be driven by a stronger need for accomplishment;
- be more dedicated to the aims of one's own occupation;
- harbor a stronger liking for the work itself; and
- have a strong need for occupational security that can be more completely met by a profession than by a job.

Overall, the professional is likely to place greater emphasis on the fulfillment of higher-order needs—the esteem needs and the need for self-actualization. In pursuit of the these largely psychological needs, the professional ordinarily

- places considerable emphasis on learning and achieving;
- prefers to do work that is interesting, stimulating, and challenging;
- desires a sense of accomplishment related to the performance of meaningful work; and
- seeks opportunities to assume responsibility and to exercise a voice in how the work is done.

Of course not all of the foregoing noble desires and actions are exhibited by every professional. A number of professionals approach work simply as many others do: as an economic means to an end. However, as it is with all employees who look for sources of motivation in the work itself, it is doubly important to do so for the professional employee. The professional employee, of all employees in the workforce, is far less likely to simply exist on a job, resigned and reasonably tolerant, merely because all environmental factors are acceptable.

By and large, the professional employee is a mover and a doer by inclination and more of a leader than a follower. The manager must recognize this in the professional, and attempt to use these characteristics in working with both the person and the job to inspire self-motivation.

Many of the better ways to arouse motivation in the professional involve the practice of open, participative management styles that promote self-control and autonomy, including the following:

- Quality circles and other forms of group problem solving
- Work simplification and other similar approaches to stimulate employee participation in the improvement of work methods
- Management by objectives (MBO) and similar approaches that are based on joint target setting
- Job enrichment approaches that expand and alter roles, perhaps including flexible hours and job rotation.

In the last analysis the true professional, dedicated to the profession and to its conscientious practice, may require only simple long-run satisfaction with environmental factors—perhaps only a tolerable environment—as long as the person's psychological needs are fully met by the work. However, even the best of environmental conditions frequently fails to hold the professional who is not receiving psychological need satisfaction from work. As suggested in Chapter 6, the unsatisfied professional is more likely than other employees to seek need satisfaction through a change of organization. This consideration calls for a brief examination of turnover among professional employees.

TURNOVER

Voluntary changes of employment are on average more frequent for the professional employee. Such changes are made in search of satisfaction of various needs, needs that are felt to an extent sufficient to make an employee abandon present employment to gain greater satisfaction. Professional employees generally know (or believe) that they can change employment more easily than others, so they are less likely to tolerate what they see as unsatisfactory conditions, and less likely to balk at stepping out into the unknown territory represented by a job change.

Difficult economic times, whether in general or within a particular industry or specific occupation, encourage people to hold onto what they have rather than seeking change as they might in better times. This is true for professionals and nonprofessionals alike; as the economy slows down, the turnover rate slows down.

The manager should always be aware that, regardless of the state of the labor market in general, professional employees are likely turnover candidates. (The exceptions are those who are unfortunate enough to be working in an overcrowded specialty.) Many professionals possess high interorganizational mobility and special skills that may well be in demand in many places. Because of this, certain approaches to management that might not cause a problem with some employees—at least no immediate turnover problem, although some other difficulties certainly arise—simply do not work for long with the mobile professional.

Bluntly stated, the professional is far less likely to tolerate the "take the job or leave it" approach, or the periodic swift-kick approach. Few if any employees ever appreciate the swift-kick approach, but those who lack the relative security of a skilled, in-demand occupation stay put and react in other ways, such as organizing into unions. At any rate, any manager who has never experienced the swift-kick approach from higher management should have learned that the propulsion provided by the kick lasts only as long as the sting from the kick. When the sting fades away, only resentment remains. The boss then discovers that the only way to get another response is to administer another kick, after which the boss often discovers that the resulting resentment is cumulative.

The manager must come to recognize that the same kinds of needs that first brought the worker into the profession—to achieve, to do interesting work, to be challenged, to do something of value, and such—are often the same kinds of needs that stimulate the professional to change organizations. This claim of the impact of professionals' psychological needs on turnover can be supported by consideration of the reasons why higher-level employees quit their jobs for new employment.

Why Valued Employees Quit

An extensive review of exit interview information acquired over a period of years led to a number of conclusions concerning why valued employees leave their jobs. Although many voluntary departures were examined, those going into the review's conclusions were limited to only resignations owing to some measure of employee dissatisfaction. Certain kinds of resignations were excluded. For example, a registered nurse leaving her position because of a spousal transfer was not counted. Many reasons for leaving were cited, but only those receiving significant multiple mentions were tabulated. This review suggested that the half-dozen primary reasons why higher-level employees leave their jobs are, in approximate order of importance:

1. **Lack of job satisfaction.** This was cited most often as the reason why people were leaving supposedly good jobs to go elsewhere. Indeed it has been established time and again that employees who are unhappy because they do not feel useful or valued, and/or who are generally dissatisfied with what they are doing, are likely to seek employment changes that appear to offer greater satisfaction.

2. **Lack of challenge.** An organization's best potential producers are usually those people who need to have the limits of their knowledge and skill tested regularly. An organization that does not make use of the full talents of its employees, and does not listen to those employees and take their suggestions seriously, tends to lose precisely those employees whom it should be most interested in retaining.

3. **Dissatisfaction with supervision.** Uncommunicative or authoritarian supervision—that is, bossism or generally authoritarian management—makes employees feel as if they are not allowed to think for themselves. A style of management that demands blind obedience and prohibits active participation eventually drives away quality employees, again precisely those employees the organization should most want to keep. Professionals especially are likely to react negatively to what they perceive as "micromanagement" by organizational superiors.

4. **Incompatibility within the work group.** This reason for leaving seems capable of surfacing at any time within any organization and at any level. It essentially involves personality clashes between people who must work together on a regular basis. Although no worker is immune to possible incompatibility, the professional, with greater interorganizational mobility, is more likely to seek active relief by changing jobs.

5. **Inadequate pay.** Opinions about the relative power of money as a motivator run the gamut from strong to inconsequential. However, many who have spent years dealing with employee complaints and administering wage and salary systems have concluded that for a great many employees money is not a significant motivator. However, the lack of money—specifically, inadequate compensation as perceived by the employee—can be a powerful dissatisfier. An organization that does not remain competitive with regard to salaries and benefits stands to lose a number of its valued employees. The notion of equity in compensation is particularly important; what is important is not so much what a person may be

paid in absolute amounts but rather what the person is paid relative to others. Money sometimes holds employees longer despite the presence of other dissatisfactions. However, if pay is the only satisfactory condition of a person's employment, it never assures contentment with employment. Some employees will of course put up with considerably undesirable circumstances if the monetary compensation is great enough. However, the money itself will not cause someone to like the job any better; it will simply encourage the person to tolerate the unsatisfactory conditions longer.

6. **Lack of confidence concerning eventual success in the job.** Employees who may feel that they are in over their heads often tend to escape that feeling by quitting and seeking employment elsewhere. The organization that fails to take active steps to develop its employees, and to demonstrate that the organization wants them to succeed, eventually loses many who could become positive contributors given the proper nurturing and support.

An Added Word about Pay

With professionals, the manager is dealing with people who are generally higher up on the need scale than the satisfaction of simply physiological and safety needs. Money remains important to most professionals, but this importance is relative to other factors. Being perhaps somewhat less concerned with the continued ability to meet all of the basic needs of life, the professional may tend to take for granted a given level of need satisfaction. Certainly in the matter of occupational or job security, basic to the safety needs, the individual may have drawn a considerable measure of need satisfaction from the process of entering the particular profession. The attitude frequently projected by the working specialist suggests a belief that the work will last, whether in one's present organization or in another. One's actions say, in effect, "I am working in my chosen field, and I always will be as long as I want to. The money could be better (could it not always be better?), but it's a good, steady income."

Employees frequently seek more money. Even those who do not actively seek more do not ordinarily refuse more money when it is granted. However, many employees, and in particular well-trained and reasonably well-paid technical and professional workers, do not necessarily seek more money for the sake of what that money can buy. Rather, to many higher-level employees money is primarily a measure of success and a form of recognition. To some professionals who bring to the workplace a drive to achieve and a competitive outlook, the paycheck stub is the "scorecard" indicating how well they are performing.

The logic is simple enough: one who learns more, grows more, accomplishes more, and takes on more responsibility is therefore worth more. In at least token fashion, a pay raise acknowledges this belief. The individual pay raise may not be particularly large, but the mere fact of its granting is often the periodic reinforcement that one may need to continue believing that one's worth is being recognized.

Professional or not, each employee desires—and expects—more money to be granted periodically even though there may not be pressing financial need in the strict sense of the word. Additional money remains far more important for what it symbolizes—recognition, reward, and reaffirmation of worth— than for what it buys.

In recalling the position of money as one of a number of environmental factors, it is essential to remember that money, although not often a true motivator, can and frequently does become a strong dissatisfier. More often than most other environmental factors, this particular factor must be reinforced periodically or its value diminishes. In other words, the employee views normal, periodic pay raises as necessary for one to stay even. Should the generally accepted period pass with no increase, this is seen as a step backward and it can provide an element of dissatisfaction.

In addition to staving off dissatisfaction and serving as a form of recognition, money frequently serves another purpose that tends to be important to many technical and professional employees: It provides an indication of how one is perceived to be regarded relative to others. At its best in this regard, money is a leveler: If employees perceive that they are equitably compensated relative to each other, they are more likely to be satisfied than if they perceive otherwise. At its worst in this regard, money is a weapon in a constant battle of one-upsmanship; one may come to regard a slightly higher level of pay as somehow affirming that one is better than another or worth more than another. At its best or at its worst, however, the effects are always present as employees continue to use salary as one of the dimensions for comparing themselves with others.

THE DEAD-END EMPLOYEE

First mentioned in the section on upward mobility in Chapter 6, the dead-end employee is the employee who has reached the highest nonmanagement position available in a given function and has for all practical purposes run out of advancement opportunity. For this person, no steps remain in the career ladder except management positions, and the person may not be considered suitable for management. (Or, management positions may become available so infrequently that this avenue of movement appears to be forever closed for all practical purposes.) There may be little or no room for horizontal movement within the organization.

An employee who has attained strict dead-end status has also topped out, that is, the person has reached the top of the salary scale for the position and can usually look forward to a pay raise only when the top of the scale is advanced. This circumstance removes much of the power of money to symbolize recognition. Instead raises, when they do come along as the scales advance, may well be seen as only a small part of one's due for tolerating the increasingly constraining conditions of one's employment.

The dead-end employee is often keenly aware of the absence of growth opportunity, and even the temporary lift provided by an occasional pay raise is likely to be dulled if not missing altogether. This employee may enjoy a far greater measure of job security than many others—the dead-end employee is usually a longer service employee, having been there long enough to move up a number of steps and advance to the top of the pay grade—but this may not be enough to stave off encroaching dissatisfaction. Job security addresses a safety need, and the person, particular the skilled professional or technical employee, eventually experiences the tug of higher-order needs.

Dead-end employees present a particular challenge for the manager. The dead-end employee is often one of the department's better employees, but dead-end status can stifle willingness and creativity and breed discontent. Money, certain benefits, and other environmental factors—all potential dissatisfiers if not periodically reinforced—may be severely limited in the dead-end situation. Certain true motivators, such as the opportunity to acquire new knowledge, may be likewise limited by the employee's prolonged exposure to the same job.

The manager must attempt to preserve the productive capability of the dead-end employee by learning how to help the employee find satisfaction in the work itself. To this end, the manager should provide the dead-end employee with the opportunity for the fulfillment of higher-order needs by

- giving the employee some decision-making responsibility whenever possible, so that the person may bring accumulated experience to bear in a way that benefits the entire department;

- delegating special one-time tasks so as to take advantage of the employee's experience and familiarity with the organization;

- using the employee to train and orient new employees;

- asking the employee for advice and suggestions, and otherwise involving the person as much as possible in determining how the work of the department is done;

- assigning prestigious projects or management of initiatives to the employee, that provide the employee with increased visibility outside the department or the organization. Examples might include representing the department or institution at certain conferences, or serving on various committees;

- using the employee as relief or backup for the manager (providing the appropriate capabilities are present); and

- giving the employee access and encouragement to attend occasional supervisory development activities, even if there may seem to be no advancement opportunity for years to come.

In general, in working with the dead-end employee the manager should be proceeding simultaneously along two tracks. First, the manager should make it possible for the employee to make a maximum contribution based on years of experience. Second, the manager should enable the employee to meet some important psychological needs.

A final word of caution regarding the treatment of the dead-end employee is in order. Frequently the manager, wishing to do something positive for a dead-end employee, attempts to have the person's position upgraded within the organization's wage and salary structure, in an effort to provide more room for movement in salary. Often the manager builds a compelling case based on the individual's vast knowledge, years of experience, and value to the organization. All of this, however, usually indicates misdirected (though well-intentioned) concern in that it is focused on evaluating the person and not the position. The manager's concern is misdirected on two counts: First, an upgrade does indeed expose the employee to a higher maximum salary and thus provides some room for movement, but the movement is limited and the problem soon resurfaces. Second, such an upgrade creates inequities within the salary structure, sets a dangerous precedent, and overall weakens the institution's wage and salary system. The effect of such an upgrade is temporary only; it simply postpones the time when an important environmental factor will become a dissatisfier. It is far better for the manager to be looking at the job itself for the means to arouse motivation in the employee.

MANAGEMENT TO MOTIVATE

In the early years of a career, the mature, serious professional who becomes dedicated to the work of the profession devotes increasingly more attention to satisfying the following needs:

- The need to do work that is interesting
- The need to experience a feeling of accomplishment from the performance of meaningful work
- The need for challenge and for the stimulation that comes with frequently testing and extending one's capacity
- The need for growth within the profession
- The need for a certain measure of recognition, status, and achievement
- The need to pursue the making of some positive contribution to the delivery of health care.

A great deal of responsibility for employee motivation rests with the manager of the professional employee. The manager must be continually aware of those things—the all-important needs—that serve as forces that bring the professional employee to work day after day. The manager must be constantly aware that the professional employee and the nonprofessional employee are probably at different levels on the hierarchy of human needs most of the time. They are likely driven by a different mix of needs, and the manager may discover that, all other factors being equal, the professional reacts more quickly than the nonprofessional to unsatisfactory conditions.

Realistically, the manager must also be aware that not everyone—professional or otherwise—demonstrates the desire, or even the capacity, to partake of the enriching, participative approaches to management that are frequently recommended as solutions to motivational problems. The frequent assumption that technical and professional employees and managers are overwhelmingly more responsive than rank-and-file employees has undermined many formal motivational programs. They may be somewhat more responsive on the average, but their numbers include many to whom work remains a means to other ends that are more important to them. True, a number of such employees may be reached readily. But a larger number of such employees are reached and motivated only with great difficulty and prolonged effort, and a surprising number are never moved at all. However, some top-management assumptions about people persist in spite of repeated experience, suggesting that such assumptions may constitute one significant area of reasons why many formal motivational programs—total quality management (TQM), management by objectives (MBO), some applications of quality circles, and the like—are doomed for failure from the start.

Although the matter of employee retention is a concern of every manager, it is of special concern to the manager of the professional. Compared with other employees, professionals are sometimes harder to find; are more difficult to recruit; may take longer to bring into the organization; may take a much longer time to develop into independently functioning workers (even though they come into the organization knowing the basics of the occupation); and usually require considerably more time, effort, and expense to replace when they leave. It is to the manager's advantage to approach the motivation of the professional employee in the full knowledge that

- the only workable way to arouse lasting self-motivation is to approach the professional employee through the work itself; and

- the first employees to leave the organization because of dissatisfaction are usually the better employees, precisely those workers whom the manager should wish to retain.

NOTES

1. A. H. Maslow, A Theory of Human Motivation, *Psychological Review* 50 (1943): 370–96.

2. F. Herzberg et al., *The Motivation to Work* (New York: John Wiley & Sons, Inc., 1969).

QUESTIONS AND ACTIVITIES

1. Provide four examples of how satisfaction of the love needs or sociological needs might be pursued both on and off the job by an individual employee.

2. Fully explain the implications of using fear and intimidation in attempting to motivate employees.

3. Explain the potential hazards inherent in upgrading a position to provide more money for an employee at the maximum of the pay grade.

4. Explain the differences between *motivators* and *dissatisfiers* by comparing and contrasting how they work and why they work (rather than simply stating what they are).

5. Where, on the Maslow hierarchy of needs, do you believe most workers reside when they are near the end of their careers? Provide reasons or hypothetical examples to support your answer.

6. Fully explain why nonprofessionals are more likely than professionals to feel a strong attachment to a particular work organization.

7. Consider a hypothetical organization in which turnover is lowest in the community, but in which average pay rates are less than those

QUESTIONS AND ACTIVITIES *(continued)*

throughout the rest of the community. Explain how this apparently contradictory condition can exist.

8. Describe the position that you believe most health care professionals enjoy in the present environment and employment market. Provide hypothetical examples to support your description.

9. Describe, with appropriate examples, how an individual might be set *backward* on the need hierarchy to lower levels, and what the immediate results of this setback might be.

10. What do you believe is the most important aspect of the proliferation and implementation of personnel policies as far as employee satisfaction and motivation are concerned? Why?

11. Express your opinion of the relative power, if any, of money as a motivator. What do you believe to be the most important question to ask relative to the attempted motivational use of money?

12. Fully explain why the more consultative and participative leadership styles are more likely than autocratic styles to work with professional employees.

13. Explain why one's compensation relative to that of others is sometimes of greater significance than one's absolute level of compensation.

14. An individual who has been out of work for some months happily accepts the first offer of employment that presents itself. Only a few months later this individual is discontented with his present employment and actively seeks another position. What can explain this person's apparently dramatic change of attitude toward his employment?

15. Describe what you believe could be done in an attempt to reinvigorate the group's most senior dead-end employee, using as an illustration a specific department or function with which you are familiar.

CHAPTER 8

Appraising the Professional's Performance

A just criticism is a commendation, rather than a detraction.
—Henry Jacob

This Chapter Will:

► Examine the possible reasons for many managers' discomfort with performance appraisal;

► Present the true objectives of performance appraisal and outline the traditional approaches to appraisal;

► Explore the validity of applying variations in the appraisal process within the same organization;

► Provide a critical analysis of performance appraisal as it is commonly practiced;

► Examine the reasons why appraisal programs often fail and outline the requirements of an effective appraisal system;

► Develop a suggested approach to the appraisal of technical, professional, and managerial employees;

► Examine the present-day legal implications of performance appraisal.

MUST APPRAISAL BE A DREADED TASK?

Many managers have come to regard performance appraisal as one of their least favorite tasks. The fact remains, though, that performance appraisal is widely considered one of the basic responsibilities of the manager. Whether or not a formal, organized system of performance appraisal exists within the organization, all managers eventually discover that they must deal with some form of appraisal because they must occasionally, or perhaps regularly, pass judgment on the performance of their employees.

For many managers, performance appraisal is difficult to come to grips with. It requires concentration and focus, and it requires time—time that may not always seem available to the manager. There are other problems, too, because it often seems as though the time in which to accomplish appraisal must be found at the expense of other activities that are perceived to be of higher priority and more immediate need. If one is involved with a system that calls for all employees to be evaluated at once, perhaps once each year or even as often as once every six months, the task looms as overwhelming and the manager may feel unable to do justice to the complete undertaking in the time available and still attend to business as usual.

Even an appraisal system that calls for employees to be evaluated on or near their anniversary dates may present problems. Under these circumstances, performance appraisal may appear as a nagging, ongoing process that is always with the manager, and the system sustains subtle but constant pressure on the manager throughout the year.

A system that requires that everyone be reviewed once a year at the same time of year may not represent the most effective approach, either. However, having made it through the annual crunch the manager can at least experience the relief of being "finished" with appraisals for 10 or 11 months to come. Under the otherwise preferable anniversary-of-hire approach, the manager may come to regard appraisal as a task that can never be completed.

The pressure placed on managers to follow the system and complete the appraisal of their employees' performance usually originates with higher management, but is transmitted by the organization's human resources department. It is usually believed that a measure of gentle pressure is required to encourage some managers to overcome their tendency to let appraisals slide. Unfortunately, because of this pressure the individual manager may come to see performance appraisal as only more paper pushed by the human resources department.

In addition to the amount of work involved, appraisal is frequently regarded as a distasteful task because of the following:

- The manager may react, either consciously or unconsciously, to the uncertainties of the appraisal system. The manager may be dealing with opinions and judgments, commodities that are rarely, if ever, absolute.

- The manager is usually aware that to apply the appraisal process properly, it may be necessary to discuss unfavorable judgments and negative observations with individual employees. The thought of this possibility is frequently discomforting.

In general, honest and thorough performance appraisal is considerably more difficult for the manager of professionals than for the manager of nonprofessionals. The less professional in nature a job may be, the more it is usually possible to be specific concerning the elements of that job. For many nonprofessional jobs one can actually see, count, or otherwise measure the output and assess quality in some objective sense. One can evaluate a number of functions on a truly objective basis in terms of whether they are completed properly, not completed, or how well they are done. In short, the structure of many unskilled and semi-skilled jobs is likely to be relatively simple and include a number of discrete, objectively measurable steps.

On the other hand the more professional a job is, the more difficult evaluation usually becomes. One may not necessarily be able to measure output with any degree of precision, and more subjectivity must be introduced into the overall process. The structure of the professional's job is less than concrete; rarely is the professional's job completely definable in a job description. (Although many have tried to define a professional's particular job, the resulting job description is often lengthy, complex, and overly detailed, and it still does not cover all contingencies.)

Recall one of the key phrases used in the so-called legal definition of a professional contained in the Fair Labor Standards Act: *the exercise of discretion and judgment.* In appraising a professional, the manager is frequently put in the position of rendering judgments on another person's exercise of judgment. Under few imaginable circumstances can the appraisal of the professional employee approach a state of precision such as a manager might wish were possible.

THE OBJECTIVES OF APPRAISAL

The primary objectives of performance appraisal should always be

- to encourage improved performance in the job that the employee presently holds;
- to provide opportunity for those employees who wish to expand their knowledge and pursue promotion and growth; and
- to provide the organization with people who are qualified for promotion as opportunities arise.

In many actively used performance appraisal systems the foregoing objectives are not well served. Many appraisal systems

- are negatively oriented, focusing primarily on criticism and faultfinding;
- remain firmly rooted in the past, failing to use the past for its only legitimate purpose: as a starting point for improvement; and
- treat the performance appraisal process as providing a snapshot, simply a static view of performance at one specific point in time.

Contrary to its use in many systems, however, the performance appraisal needs to be regarded as a process that is more positive than negative. After an appraisal has been written, the appraisal interview has been conducted, and the form has been filed, the employee should be reasonably able to answer two questions:

1. How am I doing in the eyes of my manager, and thus in the eyes of the organization?
2. What are my future possibilities?

TRADITIONAL PERFORMANCE APPRAISAL METHODS

Rating Scales

Many performance appraisal systems—probably the overwhelming majority of existing systems—use the rating scale approach. In such systems each criterion on which the employee is evaluated must be rated judgmentally on a scale that may range from totally unacceptable to perfect. Some rating scales are of the *continuous type*: A mark must be made somewhere along a continuous line drawn to represent the entire range of possible performance.

Some scales are of the *discrete* type: For a given criterion, the manager simply checks one of four, five, six, or more boxes or spaces representing gradations in performance. Such methods often include the use of points—numerical values assigned according to the position on the line of the mark or the check in a box—and the employee receives a total numerical score. Such systems often include varying weights assigned to some of the criteria. For instance, quality of work may be considered more important than appearance, and may be given two or three times the weight of appearance in the final score. Such systems may also require the manager to supply a written rationale for each score rendered, but it is the total numerical score that really indicates where the employee stands relative to management's expectations and relative to other employees.

Employee Comparison

Employee comparison methods range from informal and extremely simple to highly structured and complex. At the simple end of the scale is *ranking*, the process of judgmentally placing a small group of employees in the order of the manager's overall judgment of their capabilities. At the more involved end of the scale is a technique referred to as *forced distribution*. Forced distribution assumes a so-called normal statistical distribution of employees; that is, it uses the traditional bell-shaped curve to group employees on the assumption that the greatest number of them are average and that those who are above average and below average are equally distributed in descending order on either side of the average group.

Under the forced distribution approach, managers are usually required to distribute their employees among corridors or percentiles. One possible approach may require the manager to rate 10 percent of the employees as excellent, 20 percent as above average, 40 percent as average, 20 percent as below average, and 10 percent as unacceptable. Aside from the distinct possibility that the assumption of a normal distribution may be inappropriate to begin with, many of the inequities of this approach should be apparent.

Checklists

One method referred to as the *weighted checklist* works much like the rating scales methods, in that the manager simply checks for each performance criterion the performance level that, as judgmentally determined, appears most appropriate. The criteria are weighted, but unlike the weighting used in some rating scale systems, the actual weights applied are unknown to the manager. The weights are kept secret and are applied after the manager submits the evaluation, usually to the human resources department. This is supposedly done to prevent the manager from introducing bias into the process either intentionally or unintentionally. ("Let's see now, one notch down on quality of output is offset by two notches up on demonstrated job knowledge.") In general, however, rather than minimizing bias, the secrecy approach seems to introduce more uncertainty into the appraisal process (at least from the manager's point of view).

Another form of checklist is known as the *forced choice* method. In this method, for each evaluation criterion the manager must react to a series of statements about performance. Each group of five statements (the number most often used in such systems) includes favorable statements, unfavorable statements, and often a neutral statement. For each group of statements the manager is required to select one statement that best describes the performance of the employee and one that least describes the performance of the employee. It is felt by some that using this method to examine performance against a given criterion from both ends—the positive and the negative—helps the manager to act with minimal bias. Weights are assigned to all statements, and again these weights are usually kept secret from the manager. (At this point it may be appropriate to suggest that any performance appraisal approach that requires one or more key elements to be kept secret from the evaluators or the employees should be regarded with a highly critical eye, if not with outright suspicion.)

Critical Incident

The critical incident approach to appraisal requires that the manager keep a running log of anecdotal notes on each employee. Supposedly all critical incidents—incidents or occasions of performance that fall outside the realm of so-called normal performance either favorably or unfavorably—are recorded as they occur. Properly practiced, this system enables the manager to capture performance information when it is current. At the time of the formal review the manager simply assembles the series of anecdotal notes into a picture of the employee's overall performance for the year.

This approach is not widely used, probably because of two significant shortcomings: many employees respond unfavorably to the knowledge that their behavior is being "written up" and that much of what they do will wind up in the manager's equivalent of "the little black book"; and because manager's are busy people, they often neglect to stop what they are doing long enough to write up current incidents. Under pressure of time they tend to ignore favorable incidents and write up only the unfavorable ones, thus giving the entire process a negative flavor.

Field Review

Under the field review approach to appraisal, the manager is interviewed by a knowledgeable human resources interviewer who asks appropriate questions, listens to the manager discuss the employee's performance, and subsequently writes the performance review in narrative form for the manager's approval. It is usually necessary for the interviewer-writer to go through at least one draft, correcting and modifying what is written after reviewing it in detail with the manager.

Many managers are bound to favor this process because it requires them only to talk about the employee while someone else does the more demanding work of creating the written appraisal. However, the major drawback of this process is overwhelming: It requires an added amount of human resources department staff that few organizations of any size—especially health care provider organizations operating in today's financial environment—can afford. (Using predetermined time standards for certain kinds of work, plus a few reasonable assumptions, the human resources director of a hospital in the 400- to 500-bed range estimated that the implementation of field review for all of the hospital's employees would require the addition of at least six full-time interviewer-writers to his department.) Field review should be considered suspect to begin with—its effectiveness depends almost completely on the skill of the interviewer-writers—and from an economic point of view it should be considered inappropriate for all organizations save those with very few employees.

Free-Form Essay

The free-form essay approach requires the manager to appraise the employee by writing about the employee's performance in essay form. This approach may be somewhat structured in that the manager may be expected to cover certain specific topics in the review, perhaps including items such as job knowledge, quality of output, quantity of work, and other criteria similar to those used in other appraisal systems. As with many other appraisal approaches, doing an effective job with the free-form essay requires time and effort. Also, many people, and certainly many managers, do not regard writing as one of their favorite tasks. In addition, there is a significant flaw in this approach, in that the perceived value of a person's performance review—how "good" a review the individual may receive—may be heavily influenced by the level of the appraising manager's writing skills. A manager who can write skillfully can make an average employee appear outstanding; a manager who writes poorly can make an excellent employee appear average or even marginal.

Group Appraisal

Under the group appraisal approach an employee is reviewed, using whatever form or format may be applied, by three or four managers who are familiar with the employee's work. On the positive side, group appraisal is an excellent way to cancel potential bias because the evaluating managers must discuss each aspect of the employee's performance and come to agreement on a rating. However, if the employee is not known sufficiently well by any managers other than their own, an adequate appraisal group cannot be formed.

Peer Group Appraisal

Because it is sometimes used within a group of employees who work as an integrated team, peer group appraisal is frequently described as a form of team appraisal. Peer group appraisal is at times appropriate when a number of people work sufficiently in cooperation with each other, so that the success of any individual is largely dependent on the success of the group as a whole. This approach can be appropriate when management is attempting to build a solidly functioning team of interdependent performers. Often, individual evaluations do not facilitate team building because they do not directly address the effect of the team on the individual or the impact of the individual on the team.

Since peer group appraisal involves having the members of a team evaluate each other, it is probably most useful when used as a complement to individual appraisal rather than as a substitute for it. This approach will ordinarily reveal differences in group members' perceptions of each other.

Peer group appraisal should be as completely criteria- or competency-based as possible. Personal likes and dislikes can vary significantly within any group, thus peer group appraisal can be affected by personal bias unless the team members' subjective assessments of each other can be held to an absolute minimum.

Peer group appraisal may play an expanded role in the not-too-distant future. Mergers and other affiliations, and the trend toward decentralization that frequently accompanies them, are increasing many managers' spans of control. A manager acquiring more territory to cover and more employees to watch over may not be in a position to know all that is necessary about an individual's performance to conduct a reasonable appraisal. Therefore, peer group assessment may provide enough solid information to "fill in the blanks" for the manager.

Although a peer group appraisal is accomplished by all members of the group working together, the appraisal interview should still be a traditional face-to-face, one-on-one discussion with one's immediate manager. The manager, however, must make it clear to the employee that he or she is presenting a consensus evaluation developed by the group and not an individual assessment.

As with some of the alternative appraisal processes, peer group appraisal consumes more time than individual appraisal. Also, this process can at times be upsetting to some individuals. Appraisal leaves open the door to criticism of a sort, and not everyone will react in the same manner to criticism which represents the consensus of a number of people who are regular coworkers, and perhaps even friends. This effect can be dampened somewhat if individual observations shared within the groups are done so anonymously, but one who is criticized will always know that the commentary came from peers and not from the manager.

DIFFERENT APPROACHES FOR DIFFERENT EMPLOYEES?

No manager of an organization that utilizes a wide variety of employee skills should feel compelled to use a single appraisal approach for all employees.

However, many organizations persist in using a single appraisal process in much the same way that some people count on using stretch hosiery—one size fits all.

An approach under which all employees are reviewed with a single system is bound to be overpowering for some employees and insufficient for others. Yet many health institutions continue to use the same form, the same ground rules, and thus the same general approach for all employees, from the unskilled laborer to the highly skilled professional. A few health care organizations, however, have attempted to recognize the valid differences in appraisal approaches as related to persons in varying job grades. In some organizations, the systems in place include

- a two-system approach, evaluating nonexempt and exempt employees with different methods;

- a two-level approach that applies different evaluation criteria to management employees and nonmanagerial employees; and

- a three-system approach consisting of one set of rules for nonmanagers, one for managers, and one specific to nursing personnel.

The approach most strongly recommended herein comprises

- one system for evaluating employees who are generally nonexempt (employees who are nontechnical, nonprofessional, and nonmanagerial); and

- one system for evaluating exempt employees, that is, technical, professional, and managerial employees.

This two-system approach suggests that the organization, in developing a system specifically applicable to technical, professional, and managerial employees, is able to take appropriate advantage of the self-determining nature of professional work. Recall from the matter of the exercise of discretion and judgment, that such a system would enable a manager to provide a professional with the opportunity for individual goal setting. In short such an approach enables the manager to involve professionals in determining many of the criteria for which they will be evaluated.

Following a brief examination of some general appraisal problems, consideration turns to the identification of the elements or characteristics of an effective appraisal system. Following these considerations is the outline of one possible approach to the appraisal of professionals that embodies the preferred characteristics of an effective appraisal system.

EVALUATION OF APPRAISAL

Whether managers should appraise the performance of employees is no longer an issue, especially within the health care industry. A functioning performance appraisal system is essentially a requirement at those times when the organization is called on to defend some personnel action that it has taken. Such defenses of personnel actions are becoming increasingly necessary.

Unfortunately, some of the growing pressures on organizations encourages much appraisal to be done simply because some standard, regulation, or outside system says that it must be done. If an appraisal is accomplished simply to have it on file in case it is needed, then appraisal is being done for the wrong reasons. Many appraisals are indeed done for the wrong reasons, and frequently appraisal itself deserves a poor rating.

A particularly troublesome problem occurs in the appraisal of professionals. The appraisal of a professional by a manager who is also a professional in the same field amounts to a judgment of a peer's performance. In appraisal the manager must think and act as a manager, albeit a manager with technical knowledge. However, the professional side of the manager can readily get in the way of the process.

Most performance evaluators are considerably inexperienced in the process of evaluation and are thus unqualified, or minimally qualified, to evaluate. As with many other tasks, the more evaluations that one performs, the better one becomes at the process of evaluation. Evaluation remains an uncomfortable task, so managers tend to shy away from it. Managers perhaps encounter the necessity to evaluate only now and then and often do not get into the process long enough to gain the experience required, first, to reduce their discomfort with evaluation and, second, to improve their skill at evaluation.

Job descriptions and other job specifications are often the basis for an employee's appraisal, and if the job description is weak, then the manager begins the evaluation process partly in the dark. In the dark or not, however, managers frequently tackle performance appraisals without ensuring the presence of up-to-date job descriptions. It is important to appreciate that a true job description may exist in at least three distinctly different forms: first, in the manager's mind, as the manager's concept of how the job should be done; second, in the employee's mind, in the employee's own notion of what the job should consist of; and third, in a somewhat different form: the way it was written to begin with. If these three concepts of the job are not as close to identical as possible—and often they are considerably far apart—then it is difficult for worthwhile appraisals to be conducted.

Appraisal deserves a poor rating when it becomes apparent that the process is not generally used as an instrument to foster growth in employees and inspire positive change. Some employees may sense that appraisals are not being considered when filling newly created jobs and in making promotional decisions. These actions might be perceived as taking place according to seniority or, considerably worse, according to someone's pattern of favoritism. As a result, an employee may begin to think, What's the use of doing a good job and getting a good evaluation if it doesn't bring anything in the way or reward or recognition?

When appraisal itself is appraised, it frequently does not fare well. This is often the case because appraisal is done for the wrong reasons—perhaps to satisfy some higher management dictate, comply with the standards of certifying and accrediting bodies, or to satisfy the requirements of government agencies that deal in matters of personnel and employment.

One major effect of a requirement for performance appraisal is that it forces a manager into a certain amount of close contact with each employee. An enforced system guarantees that at least once each year the manager and employee sit down to discuss the employee's performance. However, it is unfortunate indeed if an enforced system is what is required to get the manager and employee into a face-to-face discussion of how the employee is doing, and where he or she seems to be heading. An effective manager–employee relationship is a key in the all-important business of getting things done through people. This should not have to be forced through the imposition of an appraisal system. Yet many employees in many organizations state that the only face-to-face performance-related discussions they have with their managers are their once-per-year performance appraisal discussions.

A requirement for performance appraisal alone, with its once-per-year appraisal interview, cannot establish and support an appropriate manager–employee relationship. An effective relationship requires a considerable amount of conscientious effort, primarily on the part of the manager. If the manager–employee relationship is all that it should be, then the appraisal interview becomes a mere formality because the two parties, manager and employee, know where they stand with each other at all times.

REASONS FOR APPRAISAL FAILURE

Most appraisal programs do indeed fail, or at least fall far short of their original intentions. This occurs for a number of reasons. The most significant are:

- **Ratings are based on personality judgments.** Frequently the evaluator must rate the employee using criteria that are largely indicative of personality characteristics. Exhibit 8–1 is a listing of the evaluation criteria taken from an actual appraisal system (fortunately, a system that was

Exhibit 8–1   Evaluation Criteria: Sample Appraisal System

1. Quality of work	7. Dependability
2. Volume of work	8. Attitude
3. Effectiveness	9. Cooperativeness
4 Job knowledge	10. Interpersonal relations
5. Adaptability	11. Attendance
6. Initiative	12. Appearance

abandoned and replaced some years ago). Of the 12 evaluation criteria listed, five—adaptability, initiative, dependability, attitude, and cooperativeness—are strongly rooted in personality characteristics. The criterion of interpersonal relations may be highly personality based because how one relates on the job is often tied to how one relates as an individual overall. Effectiveness may be said to have personality implications (for instance, an employee may be described as a perfectionist or a procrastinator, or as lacking the ability to see things through to the completion of all details). Even attendance and appearance are at least partial reflections of personality. By closely examining the 12 criteria one might be able to conclude that only quality of work, volume of work, and job knowledge—just 3 of 12—are relatively free of personality implications. There are also semantic problems with such rating criteria. Why is adaptability a factor? Why not consider flexibility? And how are flexibility and adaptability different, if at all? How different from each other are dependability and cooperativeness? And can attitude be expected to stand alone, or is it reflected in several of the other criteria?

The factors that are not clearly differentiated from each other are subject to the well-known halo effect. In the halo effect, the rating for one characteristic tends to influence the ratings for other characteristics in the same direction. For example, a portion (somewhat exaggerated) of a manager's thinking relative to a particular employee's performance might go as follows: "He did not respond willingly or favorably to my most recent great idea and he didn't seem able to catch on to it, so his adaptability isn't what it ought to be. He certainly did not pitch in to help implement my great idea, so his level of cooperativeness is not what it ought to be either. Because he is neither particularly adaptable nor especially cooperative, I can't say that I think much of his overall attitude." Thus the employee has lost out on three criteria through a single line of reasoning.

All of this adds up to a focus on personality, not performance. The manager is improperly encouraged to evaluate the person rather than the results of the person's efforts.

- **Evaluators are unqualified to judge.** Few managers are qualified to render personality judgments. Perhaps a manager who also happens to be a psychiatrist or clinical psychologist may be capable of rendering personality judgments. However, such managers are undoubtedly few and far between. When forced by a system to render such judgments, most managers are simply trying to do something they are not qualified to do.

- **Evaluators are discouraged from distinguishing between causes and results of behavior.** Considerable difficulties are inherent in personality-based appraisals. For example, a person who is irritable and exhibits a tendency to argue may be marked down on attitude as the manager attempts to ascribe the employee's conflicts with others as being caused by a poor attitude. However, it is the conflicts—the interpersonal problems themselves—that should be of concern, as they are the results of behavior. Unfortunately, the manager is led to second-guess the supposed cause and attempt to deal with that. Likewise, a manager may attempt to label an employee who persists in resisting change as stubborn. Once again, this amounts to an unwarranted leap from the results of someone's behavior to an attempt to assign a cause to that behavior. It is a completely unjustified leap to attempt to ascribe a personality-based cause to the results of someone's behavior. Inappropriate as this may be, though, one can understand how managers are led almost automatically to probe for cause. Most managers have been told, over and over, that when one encounters a problem, the approach to take is to identify and isolate the cause of the problem and fix it. That much is reasonable. However, the manager's problem lies in the inappropriateness of assigning cause in human personality. Looking for cause in this area assumes that the cause lies within the person. One can take steps aimed at altering the person's behavior, but one cannot do much to change the essential person. Thus most of the personality-based appraisal approach is wasted.

- **Evaluators are uncomfortable in their roles.** It is a serious matter to perform an evaluation that becomes part of a permanent record, and that can affect an individual's employment and career. Managers know this, and managers know that they have a certain amount of power over promotions, raises, and other rewards, all based on individual judgment calls. Many managers are extremely uncomfortable in this position, and they frequently compensate for this discomfort by rating many employees higher than they deserve, by rating most of their employees nearly the same as each other, or by otherwise avoiding extremes in rating so as to render the entire process harmless.

- **Few criteria are measurable in any objective sense.** Referring again to Exhibit 8–1, one should consider which, if any, of the criteria listed may be counted or measured. In truth, few of these characteristics can be measured objectively. Volume of work may be measured for some employees, and perhaps quality may be assessed by some objective means. However, even volume of work may require a largely subjective call when dealing with the self-determining professional employee, and one's judgment of quality may depend on elaborate assessment procedures. And what happens with job knowledge? Perhaps this may be tested, but who accomplishes the testing? Some employees certainly sound as though they know a great deal about the work, but as many managers and employment interviewers have discovered, the person who can *talk* a good job may not necessarily be able to *do* a good job. For many employees attendance can be counted—although perhaps not as easily for the professional employee who comes and goes without benefit of time clock or other controls. Perhaps appearance may be measured to some extent if the organization has a dress code, but dress codes are frequently vague and subject to considerable controversy. As long as systems focus on such criteria, there is little that can be effectively measured.

- **Systems are often poorly administered.** For many managers, performance appraisal is an eminently postponable process. Appraisal frequently requires a third party, such as the human resources department, to issue forms and to ride herd on timetables for the completion of appraisals. Appraisal must be kept moving, constantly nudged through the steps. The considerable amount of natural resistance to the process can cause the system to die under its own weight if it is not pushed along.

- **Follow-up on evaluations is minimal or nonexistent.** As mentioned, evaluations are frequently treated as a record of the past to be filed and forgotten. Such an attitude turns an appraisal system into a simple paper mill that specializes in producing dead records. More often that not the performance appraisal is treated like a score sheet after a game, when it should be regarded as a program for the game yet to come. The appraisal should be used as a starting point on which to build improvement. However, most of the time the last appraisal is pulled from the file only when the manager is preparing to do the employee's next appraisal. ("Let's see, what did I say about this person's attitude last time?")

REQUIREMENTS OF AN EFFECTIVE APPRAISAL SYSTEM

For a performance appraisal system to have a chance of being effective, it must meet a number of conditions. If it does not meet these conditions, the system is bound to accomplish less than expected. However, even if all of the conditions are met, success is not guaranteed.

To be effective, a system requires thorough conscientious application by managers who believe in the value of performance appraisal. Careless or indifferent application can kill even the best of systems or turn them into mere paper exercises.

The requirements of an effective appraisal system are as follows:

- **System objectives.** Overall, the system must serve the true objectives of performance appraisal as previously described.

- **System focus.** The system should focus only on performance and not on personality (a fault of many existing appraisal systems).

- **Appropriateness of criteria.** System criteria—those characteristics or requirements on which the employee's performance is evaluated—must be as appropriate as possible to the kinds of work being evaluated. Rarely does a single approach fit all jobs in a single organization, especially in a health care organization with its many and varied jobs.

- **Rationale for ratings.** The system should require verbal justification of any point ratings used. Numbers or letters may be used within the system for the sake of convenience or comparison, but each type of rating should be backed with a written rationale.

- **Employee knowledge of criteria.** Employees must know, well in advance of being evaluated, the criteria on which they will be evaluated. Ideally the criteria should relate directly to the employee's complete, current job description.

- **Management education.** Managers should be thoroughly oriented in the use of the system and thoroughly trained organization-wide in the consistent application of evaluation criteria.

- **A working tool.** Once it is completed, an evaluation should serve as a working record to be used as a starting point for monitoring progress. This is especially important with unfavorable evaluations, which should be sufficiently complete to spell out specific steps and time frames for correction and improvement.

- **Appraisal interview.** The appraisal interview should be a reality; it should not be ducked because the manager is uncomfortable, or be treated once-over-lightly or disposed of quickly because the manager feels pressed for time. The appraisal interview should be a true two-way exchange and should receive the manager's full attention for whatever time is required.

- **Self-contained record.** Once it finds a home in the employee's personnel file, a completed performance appraisal should stand on its own. No cross-reference to an appraisal manual, evaluation key, or list of explanations should be necessary in determining what any particular evaluation means.

- **System administration.** Appropriate system administration must be maintained. All scheduled review dates must be observed. Managers must receive appraisal forms and reminders at a reasonable amount of time before evaluations are due, and they must receive interim reminders to ensure that evaluations do not run late. In short, someone—usually the human resources department—needs to pay constant attention to keep the system moving.

Should any of the foregoing requirements be unsatisfied by a particular performance appraisal system, the system will fall short of its full potential.

A SUGGESTED APPROACH

A thorough approach to the appraisal of the performance of the professional employee is one that

- eliminates significant reliance on personality judgments;

- bases a significant part of the evaluation on performance against a comprehensive job description; and

- bases a significant part of the evaluation on criteria that are established with the involvement and participation of the employee.

The following approach refers to three related exhibits:

- Exhibit 8–2 is a simple form that can be used for rating an employee relative to his or her job description.

- Exhibit 8–3 briefly describes the appraisal ratings that the evaluator would use when completing the Performance Appraisal–Part 1.

- Exhibit 8–4 is a simple form to be used in the participative phase of the performance appraisal.

Exhibit 8–2   Performance Appraisal–Part 1

		AVERAGE SCORE

NAME	TITLE	REVIEW DATE
DEPARTMENT	APPRAISER'S NAME	APPRAISER'S SIGNATURE

COMMENTS

Job Duty Number	Numeric Score	

COMMENTS ON POLICY ADHERENCE

ASSESS EMPLOYEE'S CAPABILITY OF ASSUMING ADDITIONAL RESPONSIBILITIES AND/OR POTENTIAL FOR PROMOTION AS APPROPRIATE

EMPLOYEE COMMENTS (To be entered by the Employee, if desired)

APPRAISER'S INITIALS	DATE	SIGNATURE ACKNOWLEDGES RECEIPT OF THIS FORM	EMPLOYEE'S SIGNATURE	DATE

COMMENTS (Appraiser or others as appropriate)

SIGNATURE AND DATE BY NEXT HIGHER LEVEL OF MANAGEMENT, THEREBY INDICATING CONCURRENCE WITH QUALITY AND CONTENT	SIGNATURE	DATE

Exhibit 8–3   Part 1 Appraisal Ratings

---

1. Unsatisfactory: unable to meet job requirements; performance not acceptable

2. Marginal: occasionally produces results that are less than required; regularly requires more than normal supervision

3. Standard: regularly performs all duties satisfactorily under normal supervision; the performance of a trained, fully functioning employee

4. Above standard: occasionally exceeds job requirements; always performs at least at standard and sometimes better

5. Well above standard: consistently exceeds job requirements, producing superior results most of the time

6. Exceptional: performance rarely achieved by others; highest possible level of performance

---

Performance Appraisal–Part 1

This is essentially a rating scale evaluation in that a numeric score is associated with each of a number of criteria. However, this approach differs from many rating scale approaches in that the criteria used are the employee's major work responsibilities as spelled out in the job description. For each major job duty in the job description, the evaluator applies a score, as appropriate, using the appraisal ratings in Exhibit 8–3. In applying such ratings one cannot help but become caught up in the making of subjective judgments, especially when dealing with professional employees for whom many legitimate job description elements are not such that performance against them can be measured in any absolute sense. Because the essence of professional work involves the exercise of discretion and judgment, it falls to the manager to determine how well the employee applies discretion and judgment in work. However, in basing the ratings strictly on the elements of a comprehensive job description, the manager is at least limiting the application of judgment to job performance, and is avoiding the problems raised by personality judgments.

In the Performance Appraisal–Part 1, the employee's average score is determined simply by adding up the individual scores and dividing by the total number of scores. This approach is sufficiently flexible that, if in the manager's judgment one or two particular job duties are considerably more important than others, the average score may be weighted to favor the more important elements. For example, if job duty 1 is considered twice as important as all other job duties, then the score for job duty 1 is added in twice when determining the average score.

Exhibit 8–4   Performance Appraisal–Part 2

Codes: (A) Complete, or progress above satisfactory
(B) Progress satisfactory
(C) Progress behind schedule

Date of Last Review

WORK IMPROVEMENT EVALUATION

Goal No. Set In Last PAIR	CODE	COMMENTS

Employee's Signature	Supervisor/Manager's Signature	Date

GOAL SETTING

Goal Number		DESCRIPTION OF GOAL

Next scheduled review	Employee's Signature	Supervisor/Manager's Signature	Date

The section for comments on policy adherence allows the manager to record any information deemed helpful or necessary concerning how the employee observes those requirements placed on all members of the organization's workforce. Because compliance with certain work rules is expected of all employees, and because disciplinary action may be based at least in part on the compliance record that the employee is establishing, it may be especially helpful to summarize the employee's observance of such requirements. This space may prove helpful for capturing information about the employee's attendance record. For instance, should an employee be approaching the organization's limit regarding tardiness or absenteeism, that information—objectively, in terms of numbers of times and perhaps even dates—should be captured here.

There is a space in which the manager is asked to assess the employee's capability of assuming additional responsibilities, or otherwise to assess the employee's potential for promotion; that is, a brief assessment of the overall potential of the employee. At the time an appraisal is completed, the manager may see no additional responsibilities that the employee could assume, and there may be no apparent promotional opportunities in existence or on the horizon. However, recognition of the employee's potential provides positive reinforcement for the employee, and also serves to help the organization identify people who may be capable of moving up as opportunities arise.

A thorough performance appraisal should include the opportunity for the employee to comment on the evaluation if desired. It is certainly not essential that an employee comment on the appraisal (many employees rarely, if ever, do so). However, it is important that this opportunity be available to employees.

As is usually the case with most performance appraisals, the Performance Appraisal–Part 1 calls for the employee's signature. This signature is requested at the end of the performance appraisal interview, following the manager's explanation to the employee of, first, the opportunity for the employee to enter comments if desired and, second, the clear understanding that the employee is not signing to indicate agreement with the appraisal but is rather signing to acknowledge that the appraisal occurred and that the employee has received a copy. An employee who disagrees with any aspect of an appraisal should be encouraged to note that disagreement under employee comments before signing the appraisal form. A space is also provided for comments by the appraiser or by others as appropriate. (The "others" are primarily the next highest level of management, as such persons are often expected to review the appraisals performed by their subordinate managers.)

Part 1 Appraisal Ratings

A review of the language describing the six levels of appraisal rating that may be used in this approach might raise a number of questions about meaning. This is understandable because what is, for example, unsatisfactory or exceptional may vary from evaluator to evaluator. A number of common problems exist in all systems in which performance rating scores are tied to word descriptions of performance: words have different meanings to different people, and rarely is one evaluator's notion of a given performance description exactly the same as another evaluator's notion.

However, one word that is commonly applied in many appraisal approaches is deliberately avoided in this approach. That word is *average*. Many performance appraisal approaches go forth under the assumption that *average* and *standard* are essentially the same. This simply is not true. The *average* performance of a given work group may be either more or less than what is expected as standard performance. One would hope that through the process of conscientiously applying the requirements of probationary periods and working to develop employees, after a time the average performance of a work group would stand at something above standard because the substandard performers have been weeded out while others have been encouraged to grow.

The key to the application of the Part 1 appraisal ratings lies in the final phrase of the sentence describing rating 3 ("standard"): *the performance of a trained, fully functioning employee.* The spread of ratings above the standard is simply a matter of thinking downward and upward on either side of that standard, considering *unsatisfactory* as just that—performance not acceptable—and *exceptional*, for all practical purposes, as nearly perfect.

Performance Appraisal–Part 2

This form can be used to address the participative part of the suggested process. The lower half of the form is used to address work improvement goals that the employee has agreed to pursue. The upper half of the form is used to record the manager's evaluation of the progress against work improvement goals previously established. The specific format of the performance appraisal is unimportant; what is important is that a record of work improvement goals and evaluation of progress against those exist in writing. A simple memo format would serve the purpose fully as well.

With the foregoing in mind, it is appropriate to examine how all the pieces can be made to fit together in a positive performance appraisal approach that is geared specifically to higher-level employees (primarily professional, technical, and managerial employees). The following steps are part of the suggested approach.

Job Description Review and Update

If an evaluator is to base a significant part of an employee's evaluation on the employee's job description, the job description must be as complete and current as possible. Further, the specific content of the job description must be known and agreed to by both employee and manager. The job description review and update should proceed as follows:

- Working alone, the employee thoroughly analyzes the job description and develops the best possible determination of how and in what ways the job description should be revised. The employee should attempt to make the job description as complete as possible relative to what should be done, and further should attempt to establish priorities for major job duties. Overall, the employee should be attempting to express on paper the complete, up-to-date concept of the structure of the job.

- Completely separate from the employee's initial activity, the manager should likewise go through the job description in detail, performing essentially the same steps that the employee is performing. The manager should likewise be attempting to portray the concept of that particular job as it is presently envisioned.

- When employee and manager have completed their independent job description analyses, they should negotiate complete agreement on a final job description. In addition to reaching agreement on the content of the job, they should arrive at agreement on the relative importance of the major job responsibilities. For that matter, the entire process should focus on describing the employee's job in a few—perhaps five, six, or seven— areas of job responsibilities. One or two of these areas of responsibilities must admittedly be catchall areas; however, in terms of being able to use a job description in any realistic sense for performance appraisal, it would hardly pay to list numerous specific tasks that occur only infrequently and require only a small amount of time. For example, a job description requirement of the employee to serve on the institution's safety committee is not worthy of separate enumeration if it only requires attendance at one meeting every three months. Such an item is better captured under a blanket statement referring to the performance of certain support functions. Once the job description has been completely brought up to date through the joint efforts of the employee and the manager, it may be used as the basis for the employee's performance appraisal.

Initial Part 1 Appraisal

Using the Part 1 appraisal ratings described in Exhibit 8–3, the manager completes the Performance Appraisal–Part 1 based on the updated job description.

The manager invites the employee to a private performance appraisal interview scheduled with at least a modest amount of advance notice (perhaps one working week). In conducting the interview the manager should review each rating applied to each job duty and explain the reasons for the evaluation. The Performance Appraisal–Part 1 form allows room for comments in support of each rating. These should be used at all times because a numeric score alone tells the employee little about the manager's assessment of performance. In the process of the appraisal interview the employee should be allowed significant time to talk about each rating and should be encouraged to do so. During this discussion the employee and manager should attempt as much as possible to work out differences that may arise in how one may see a given rating relative to how the other sees it. If differences are successfully reconciled, all is well and good. If the interview ends and differences remain, the employee should be encouraged to state this in the employee comment section of the form.

This step—the appraisal interview—helps establish the framework for subsequent steps that lead to the second part of the performance appraisal. An additional activity that might be helpful as part of this step is a self-appraisal by the employee. The manager who favors the use of self-appraisal by the employee should consider doing so only if the employee agrees to participate in a self-appraisal. Regardless of how openly the process may be approached, any number of employees may feel considerably uncomfortable with appraising themselves. However, if an employee readily agrees to a self-appraisal— and simply goes through a Performance Appraisal–Part 1 using himself or herself as the subject—then employee and manager ordinarily increase their chances of making the appraisal interview a highly constructive session. It is true that the occasional employee uses the self-appraisal as an opportunity for an ego trip and submits unjustifiably high self-ratings. However, the majority of employees can be counted on to examine their own performance critically, and more often than not an employee self-appraisal is less favorable than the evaluation rendered by the manager.

Consider, for example, the appraisal of an employee with a job description that has seven major job duties or areas of responsibility. If the interview is based only on an appraisal done by the manager, the two parties may have to talk about all seven task areas to an extent at least sufficient to identify those aspects of performance on which the manager and employee may not completely agree.

However, if the employee with seven major job duties has done a self-evaluation and the scores for five of the seven items are nearly the same as the scores given by the manager, then the two parties know immediately that their discussion must focus on the two remaining areas of performance. Overall, the self-appraisal can be extremely valuable in helping employees feel that they have an active part in the evaluation process.

Target Setting

For this part of the process the employee should be supplied with the form Performance Appraisal–Part 2.

Once again working alone, the employee should draft a plan of perhaps five or six targets to pursue for self-improvement. These performance targets, or objectives, may cover any aspect of job performance. The manager should not dictate objectives at all as far as the specific shape they take is concerned; however, the manager should go as far as advising the employee that the objectives must in part address any job responsibilities which were graded below 3 (i.e., less than standard) on the Performance Appraisal–Part 1.

In preparation for this step, the manager need give some thought only to the specific kinds of objectives that the employee might be expected to adopt in order to address areas of substandard performance, and be prepared to recommend (but never to dictate) such objectives to the employee if the employee does not specifically address such needs in his or her plan of objectives.

When both parties are prepared, they should work together—once again in a spirit of negotiation—to arrive at a set of employee objectives. These objectives should be both appropriate in addressing the employee's needs for performance improvement and consistent with the needs and objectives of the department. The manager's role in this process should be primarily that of counselor, ensuring, first, that as far as possible each of the employee's objectives is realistic and attainable, and that each objective embodies a statement of what, how much, and when. For example, "To reduce billing errors from my section" is weak because it includes only one element (the *what*) of an appropriate objective. Rather, an appropriate expression of this objective might read: "To reduce billing errors coming out of my section (*what*) by 50 percent (*how much*) within six months (*when*)."

As part of the process of negotiating objectives, the manager and the employee should be certain that they are in agreement on the *when* of each objective, and should also agree as to when they will jointly examine results. Not all objectives can be accomplished within the same time frame. Some objectives may take six months or less; others might require a year and a half to two years to attain. The objectives and their agreed-upon time frames should be captured in the goal-setting portion of the Performance Appraisal–Part 2.

Follow-up Appraisal

It is important to stress that the follow-up appraisal—the assessment of the employee's performance in pursuing specific objectives—should be done at various times throughout the year and not necessarily only when the Performance Appraisal–Part 1 is accomplished. The primary appraisal is on a regular cycle, ordinarily occurring once per year. However, the time frames for specific objectives pursued by the employee may run anywhere from six months or less to two years or more. It is most appropriate to perform a work improvement evaluation relative to the objectives expressed on Performance Appraisal–Part 2 at a more frequent interval, preferably three or six months. At the time of this interim appraisal the employee's performance in pursuit of his or her goals is evaluated. Some goals may be attained; some goals may have to be adjusted based on current information; and perhaps progress may have accrued against certain other goals and should be noted.

The essentially ongoing Performance Appraisal–Part 2 keeps the manager and the employee in regular constructive contact regarding the employee's performance. Also, the information gained through the Part 2 appraisal provides the manager with a head start in preparing for the next regularly scheduled Part 1 appraisal. When it is time for the formal Part 1 appraisal, it becomes a simple matter to refer to the current Part 2 appraisal to determine where the employee appears to be heading relative to items that may have been marginal or substandard on the previous formal appraisal.

Regular Review and Update

At least once per year the manager and the employee should reexamine the employee's job description and see that it is updated as necessary. Unless a job description has changed considerably because of outside factors (e.g., extensive rearrangement of duties among employees, the introduction of new equipment or new technology), the annual update of a job description should be a relatively simple matter.

Overall, what has been described represents a combination of activities that bring the manager and the employee together regarding the employee's performance. There is, first, the regular annual cycle that involves a reexamination of the job description and an assessment of the employee's performance.

Second, and ongoing with the steps in the regular cycle, the manager and employee should examine progress toward objectives that have been set in anticipation of improved performance. Overall, this suggested approach accomplishes the following:

- When afforded proper system administration, thorough management training, and conscientious management practice, the recommended technique can fulfill all of the requirements of an effective appraisal system.

- It bases an employee's evaluation solidly on job performance.

- It permits maximum employee participation, a condition important for professional employees.

- It encourages the manager and employee to work together and thus strengthens the manager–employee relationship

- It orients the major emphasis of performance appraisal toward future guidance and away from simple recording of the past.

The intent of the suggested approach may be summarized as follows: From the manager's perspective, it ensures that the employee is encouraged to perform at least at standard in all areas of job responsibility. From the employee's perspective, it provides the opportunity for innovation in striving for above-standard performance through the pursuit of personally determined objectives.

LEGAL IMPLICATIONS OF PERFORMANCE APPRAISAL

Unfortunately, performance appraisal brings with it a steadily increasing number of potential legal traps for both evaluator and organization.

Many lawsuits alleging wrongful termination are an outgrowth of inadequate performance appraisal processes, or appraisal processes that are poorly administered. Wrongful discharge complaints have been increasing for several years, and performance appraisal records are invariably key elements in addressing such complaints. In the majority of states, personnel policy manuals and employee handbooks have been found in the courts to constitute forms of employment contract. In many instances these documents either promise or imply that one may expect continued employment in exchange for acceptable performance, so when one is terminated in spite of a record of "good performance" the conditions are set for a charge of wrongful discharge.

The majority of legal complaints related to performance appraisals involve violations of individual rights directly provided by Title VII of the Civil Rights Act of 1964 and the Civil Rights Act of 1991. Other applicable laws often cited in claims of unlawful discharge include the Age Discrimination in Employment Act, the Americans with Disabilities Act, the Family and Medical Leave Act, and the Pregnancy Discrimination Act. Frequently, two or more laws will be cited within a single charge. For example, an older worker who claims to have been forced into unwanted retirement because of age may cite both the Civil Rights Act of 1964 and the Age Discrimination in Employment Act.

There no doubt are some who will suggest that a performance appraisal system is unneeded, pointing out that the organization is not legally required to have such a system. The health care organization, however, is subject to the accreditation requirements of the Joint Commission on Accreditation of Health Care Organizations (JCAHO) and regulatory requirements of state health agencies. It may not have the full force of law, but the organization must have a performance appraisal process in place (and satisfy numerous other requirements as well) to acquire and maintain JCAHO accreditation, and must have JCAHO accreditation to be able to receive government third-party reimbursement (mainly Medicare and Medicaid) for rendering services. Thus from the organization's perspective, the requirement for a performance appraisal system might as well be a law.

Organizations that do not fall under such accreditation and regulatory requirements are not legally required to have an appraisal system. However, *if* such an organization does have an appraisal system those external agencies that deal with employee complaints will insist that the system be applied fairly and consistently.

Although some states still retain employment-at-will status—that is, some states have laws proclaiming that the employment relationship may be ended at any time by employer or employee whether for cause or not—for all practical purposes any termination can be challenged externally. And any instance in which termination involves performance issues may send external agencies—and the courts—into the organization's personnel files for a look at performance appraisals.

For example, when a layoff occurs, management might wish to cut staff in a rational manner that eliminates poorer performers while retaining better performers. When one is terminated for performance reasons and the termination is challenged, there had best be performance appraisals on file backing up management's complaints about performance.

Significant problems have been known to arise from lenient appraisals. Consider the manager who claims to have finally "had it" with a particular employee—always a poor performer, uncooperative, often late, and never really a team player—and wants this person discharged. Now. But a survey of the individual's personnel file reveals nothing but several years' worth of "satisfactory" evaluations. In brief, when an employee is terminated for reasons of inadequate performance there had better be confirming information in the personnel file. And the best confirming information available is often thorough, well-documented performance appraisals.

IN PERSPECTIVE

To some extent the manager may always be uncomfortable with appraisal and may never be completely certain of making all the correct moves with complete justification. However, some measure of discomfort with the process is acceptable for two reasons:

1. This discomfort—and it may be no more than a vague, ill-defined uneasiness with the process—acknowledges the importance of the appraisal process. The manager should always be aware that he or she is dealing with information that is extremely important to the employee and that can have long-lasting impact.

2. Even the best performance appraisal approaches require a certain amount of subjectivity on the part of the manager in rendering judgments about the employee's performance. The manager must recognize the weaknesses inherent in human judgment and appreciate that these judgments may affect the employee's career.

Should the material covered in this chapter seem indicative of an involved, time-consuming process, that's because more often than not it is. The business of developing employees and helping them improve their performance is one of the most important tasks of the manager. Many of the higher-order needs of employees—among them appreciation of work done, knowledge of the results of one's efforts, participation and input in determining the form and structure of one's job, work that is interesting and stimulating, and the opportunity for promotion and growth—are relatively strong needs in the majority of professional employees. These and other higher-order needs are served in part through the conscientious application of effective performance appraisal.

QUESTIONS AND ACTIVITIES

1. Describe what you believe is the principal problem associated with the use of subjective assessments in performance appraisal.

2. Explain what you believe—if anything—is the primary shortcoming of the appraisal approach referred to as "forced distribution."

QUESTIONS AND ACTIVITIES *(continued)*

3. Take a position in favor of either all-at-once appraisal or anniversary date appraisal and provide in detail the reasons for your choice.

4. Provide an example of a job for which performance appraisal could be relatively simple, objective, and accurate, and explain why such an appraisal is possible in this instance.

5. Consider the situation of an employee who is by all appearances contented with the job he has worked for many years, is consistently performing well, and will clearly never be able to rise further in the organization. Why bother evaluating this employee's performance on a regular basis?

6. Describe in some detail how you would approach the appraisal of an employee who works an overlapping shift, such that you see her less than two hours per day and she works alone most of the time.

7. Fully explain why it is recommended that an employee's sign-off be obtained on a performance appraisal at the time of the appraisal conference.

8. Explain why performance appraisal is frequently viewed negatively by managers and employees alike.

9. Explain why the human resources department's role in overseeing the organization's performance appraisal system is both legitimate and necessary.

10. Take a position either for or against tying the amount of an individual's pay increase to the person's performance appraisal score. Fully explain your reasoning.

11. Explain why managers are frequently advised against reviewing an employee's previous appraisal before writing a current appraisal.

12. Describe how you would proceed with an employee who vehemently objects to the contents of his performance appraisal and who refuses to sign the appraisal.

13. Take a position either for or against making self-appraisal a required part of your organization's appraisal system, and fully explain your position.

QUESTIONS AND ACTIVITIES *(continued)*

14. Explain why this book and other references strongly advise against personality-based appraisal and why it is generally inappropriate to appraise on characteristics such as "attitude."

15. Explain why it is important to use specific instances of behavior rather than general descriptions of behavior in appraising performance.

16. Explain why it is recommended that a written rationale be provided to accompany each rating "score" that is entered in a performance appraisal.

17. Describe the likely reasons why a great many rating-scale appraisal systems use an odd number of scale points (e.g., three, five, or seven).

18. Describe what you believe is essentially wrong with appraisal systems for which certain criteria weights or calculation methods are kept secret from evaluators.

19. Describe what you believe to be the strongest advantage of peer group appraisal, and cite the circumstances under which you believe this appraisal process should be considered.

20. Regarding updating a job description in preparation for appraisal, why involve the employee in this process? The manager is ultimately responsible for the department's output, so why shouldn't the manager update the job description unilaterally?

CHAPTER 9

Day-to-Day Management of the Professional Employee

How do you spot a leader? They come in all ages, shapes, sizes, and conditions. Some are poor administrators, some are not overly bright. One clue: Since most people per se are mediocre, the true leader can be recognized because, somehow or other, his people consistently turn in superior performances.

—Robert Townsend

This Chapter Will:

► Discuss the professional employee as a sometime scarce resource, suggesting a necessary focus on retention.

► Introduce the high-skill professional and review the special management problems involved in directing such personnel.

► Outline the occasional problems encountered concerning the manager's credibility with the professional employee.

► Discuss several aspects of day-to-day management in which the manager must put more into the manager–employee relationship, or perhaps act in a particular way, because the employee is a professional.

► Establish the manager's critical role as the essential link between an employee's profession and the rest of the health care organization.

THE PROFESSIONAL AS A SCARCE RESOURCE

Oversupply and Undersupply

In the past several decades, many health care specialties have experienced conditions of oversupply. On the other hand, on numerous occasions many parts of the country have experienced shortages of certain skills, and organizations have been forced to compete for the services of available workers. Once a department's personnel needs are met, though, the focus of the manager—and certainly much of the focus of the organization's human resources department—should turn from recruitment to the important matter of retention. In short, when potential employees of certain critical skills are scarce, it is necessary to concentrate on keeping the people who are already in the organization.

A brief assessment of the supply of and the demand for various health care professionals during these early years of the twenty-first century suggests that conditions of oversupply are likely to be few and far between, while shortages have become chronic and widespread. It has become increasingly difficult for many health organization department managers to meet and maintain all of their personnel needs. As a result, instead of shifting their focus from recruiting to retention they find that both concerns are ongoing. In short, the manager of today's health care professional must be vigilant in terms of both recruiting and retention needs. Attempting to manage these mobile, much-in-demand workers provides an additional challenge, as for a number of reasons they are more difficult to manage than ever before.

Consider, for example, professional nurses. The management of professional nurses, especially in the setting of the acute-care hospital, has in recent years become increasingly complex. Financial restrictions, technological innovations, professional labor unions, and the changing attitudes of nurses are having a considerable impact on the practice of nursing. In many parts of the country the recruitment of professional nurses has become highly competitive. Health care employers are, in their attempts to fill their patient care needs, competing with other employers to hire from a nursing pool that is not growing at anywhere near the rate at which demand is increasing. The recruitment of professional nurses has become highly competitive, and it is likely to remain that way for some time.

The Increasing Importance of Retention Efforts

The retention of professional nurses is emerging as one of the most challenging tasks ever faced by health care administrators. Where once it was possible to accept relatively high turnover among professional nurses—after all, it was recognized that many nurses entered or left the work force practically at will, and there were always more available to take their places—organizations have been finding their sources of help drying up. As a result, they have had to turn their attentions partially to reducing turnover while continuing to recruit aggressively. Thus attention shifts naturally to factors and conditions that have a bearing on job satisfaction, such as better pay scales, more generous benefits, more attractive personnel schedules, additional compensation for generally less popular assignments, a more clearly defined role for the professional nurse, and a stronger nursing voice in matters of patient care.

Generally, the health care organization should wish to retain employees who are functioning satisfactorily, but the organization may not be inclined to do any more about retention than has already been done as long as replacement employees are available. However, when a given specialty is in short supply, an organization should do what can be done to retain those skilled employees —but always within limits. To take steps that are perceived as favoring one group or class of employees over others is to invite trouble; what is done for one group is frequently done for other groups as well. There are costs associated with active retention efforts because factors like improved benefits and generous staffing patterns certainly cost money. For specialties in short supply, however, the cost of retaining employees is not nearly as high as the ongoing cost of continually recruiting, hiring, orienting, and training replacements. It is true that some professionals may be considered scarce resources because of their limited numbers. However, it behooves the manager to consider *all* steadily and satisfactorily functioning employees—professional or otherwise—as equally worthy of the organization's best retention efforts.

THE HIGH-SKILL PROFESSIONAL: SOME SPECIAL MANAGEMENT PROBLEMS

The High-Skill Professional in the Health Care Organization

The high-skill professional has usually undergone extensive education, frequently possessing a master's degree or perhaps a doctorate (medical or otherwise), and is likely to be employed in a position that entails a great deal of operating autonomy. The high-skill professionals found working in or for a hospital might include the following:

- A physician or dentist employed by the hospital;
- A professional administrator engaged to operate the hospital or to run one of the hospital's major subunits;
- A certified public accountant engaged to audit the hospital or perhaps employed to manage the institution's finance division;
- A chemist or physicist engaged in research or in day-to-day operations; and
- A management consultant engaged to solve a problem for the hospital.

Such persons have two obvious characteristics in common: they are extensively educated, and they are on their own much of the time in the performance of their work.

The high-skill professional often presents the manager with some special problems and unique challenges. Frequently these problems and challenges exist because of some of the same factors that contribute to the professional's ability to perform as desired.

Characteristics of the High-Skill Professional

The high-skill professional may generally be described by some or perhaps all of the following:

- As are many employees, the high-skill professional is accountable for results. However, this person is primarily responsible for getting things done and then later, if at all, reporting the results. There is only limited or occasional need for clearing actions or decisions in advance. In this regard, the high-skill professional possesses a significant degree of operating autonomy.

- The high-skill professional may have a great deal of geographic mobility, ranging throughout an entire facility, or, as in the case of a management consultant or an auditor, from organization to organization and even from city to city.

- Being a solitary operator much of the time, the high-skill professional must consistently exercise discretion and judgment.

- The successful high-skill professional general exhibits a high degree of self-confidence and independence of thought and action.

- The successful high-skill professional appears as a self-starter who is also highly self-sufficient in work performance. The high-skill professional is able to function with minimal supervision for direction, at times for prolonged periods.

Additional examples of high-skill professionals and their operating environments are as follows:

- Visiting nurses and numerous other public health professionals who travel to visit their clients or patients, and who normally work alone;

- Hospital association staff consultants who either individually, or in small teams, travel to serve any number of member institutions in various professional capacities;

- Physicians or other scientists engaged in individual research; and

- A group of biomedical engineers who provide medical equipment service to several hospitals in a consortium.

In general, the high-skill professional is a highly educated specialist who largely operates independently, determining what needs to be done and often doing it without direct management. However, many characteristics that make for an effective high-skill professional also tend to make that employee difficult to manage at times. This is especially true of the characteristics related to independence—those factors that make an individual an effective lone operator. It is certainly important to cultivate independence in those persons who are on their own much of the time. However, at times even the lone operator must be counted on to be a team player. This is especially true when there are changes in policy and practice that may have effects on how the professional operates.

Some might say that one must also have a healthy ego to be able to presume to operate in a mode that can often be described as that of the visiting expert. The high-skill professional is indeed one who may often be viewed as needing to be in control of the situation. The healthy ego, so helpful to the professional while on assignment, can sometimes be troublesome to the manager.

In brief, this high-skill professional should ideally be

- sufficiently independent to work alone most of the time, and yet willing to respond to management direction when necessary;

- sufficiently confident to deal willingly with a wide range of problems and yet be able to subordinate the ego in dealings with management; and

- willing to accept sole responsibility most of the time, and yet be able to become a team player when the occasion demands.

The High-Skill Professional and the Manager

The manager of the high-skill professional must:

- Be thorough and cautious in the recruitment and selection process, ensuring that basic educational requirements have been met and that all necessary credentials are present and in order. For a job candidate with experience, the manager should look for a demonstrated record of success and for sound, logical reasons for wishing to make a change. For a newly graduated professional, academically qualified but inexperienced, the manager should look for self-confidence and a strong desire to do that particular kind of work.

- Try to learn what it is that most strongly motivates the individual. Often the effective high-skill professional has a strong liking for the work and a strong desire for achievement and accomplishment. The best independently functioning professionals like the work, are driven to do the work their own way, and have a great need to see the results of their efforts.

- Pay close attention to the orientation of the new employee, initially teaming the new hire with the most successful or experienced employee in the department. Even the well-experienced professional, when new to this particular organization, needs to be thoroughly oriented to the organization and its policies and people before being turned loose to function independently. After basic administrative orientation, the manager should allow the new hire growing independence by assigning tasks of increasing scope and responsibility.

- In addition to knowing the rules and policies of the organization, make certain that the new hire knows the results expected from each assignment. The manager should take care to define thoroughly the boundaries for independent action, such that the individual is able to develop a sense for how much may be done independently and when it is necessary to call for management assistance.

- Once the boundaries for management action are established, give the professional complete freedom to operate within those boundaries. The manager must strive to develop trust in the individual, and in reflecting this trust endeavor to instill in this person the belief that management has confidence in his or her ability. The manager must not violate the boundaries described by trying to dictate from afar; besides often not working, absentee management serves only to frustrate the employee. In evaluating the performance of this high-skill professional, it is essential that the manager focus most strongly on the individual's degree of achievement of expected results. The manager should leave the individual as much freedom as possible in determining how the expected results will be pursued. The manager should also consider basing performance appraisals at least in part on the achievement of objectives established with the employee's participation (joint target setting, a process similar to management by objectives but applied primarily to nonmanagerial employees).

- Finally, introduce changes—whether changes in policies, practices, operating guidelines, equipment, or whatever—with plenty of advance warning. If at all possible, the manager should allow and even encourage the employee to take part in determining the scope and direction of each change.

In summary, a number of characteristics that make a high-skill professional an effective employee may also at times make the person difficult to manage. On the one hand, independence and self-confidence must be encouraged; on the other hand, the same characteristics must be not be allowed to develop to a point at which the manager no longer has any influence on the employee's behavior. The manager is most likely to succeed with the high-skill professional by applying an open, participative management approach that gives the employee a clear, strong voice in determining how the work is done.

CREDIBILITY OF THE PROFESSIONAL'S SUPERIOR

When there are professional employees in a work group, there is always the potential for questions about the manager's credibility with those employees. There is always the potential for differences of professional opinion, and there is always the likelihood of varying degrees of unwillingness of the professional employee to accept direction from the manager.

Whether such credibility problems and their attendant difficulties exist in a given work group depends on the background and qualifications of the employees. Problems arise from the presence of a certain amount of ego, and the belief that one's profession is at least a bit more important than other occupations. Some problems arise from a sense of territorialism exhibited by many professionals; the belief that no one should hold sway over any aspect of professional performance without being on the inside.

Management credibility problems may exist when the manager is not of the same profession as the individual employee. For example, the director of nursing service who is a registered nurse may not be viewed or responded to in the same way by an employee who is a registered nurse, one who is qualified as a nurse practitioner, and perhaps one who is a certified nurse anesthetist. Similarly, an employed physician may question the credibility of an administrative superior who is a professional administrator, or perhaps who has stepped into administration from dentistry. Likewise a professional trained as a chemist may have problems relating to an immediate superior whose background is that of a medical technologist. In all such cases there may be tendencies to differ on professional judgments. ("He is only a medical technologist—who is he to tell me what I should be doing as a chemist?") There may be feelings of territorialism. ("Chemistry is my area, and only a chemist can legitimately make judgments that involve chemistry.")

Credibility problems are also likely to arise when the manager is perceived as limited to a lower professional level than the employee. Thus, the clinical psychologist with a doctoral degree may be less than completely willing to accept the leadership of a manager whose education stopped at the master's degree level; and the certified public accountant may balk at the direction of a managing accountant who is not similarly certified. It again becomes a matter of one person, the "higher" professional, being unwilling to accept the judgment of another person, the manager, who happens to be "lower" on the professional scale. In such situations there are also more hints of territorialism, as there appear to be more exclusive territories within the broader territories that are mentally reserved for those of greater status.

Problems of management credibility are highly likely in situations in which employees see their managers as nonprofessionals. To understand such credibility problems fully, one must appreciate that many individual professionals do not regard management as a profession in its own right. There are occasional organizational relationships in which a nonmanagerial professional must report directly to a nonprofessional. In one organization, for example, a registered record administrator (R.R.A.) and a utilization review coordinator who was a registered nurse reported to a director of health information management, who was a management generalist and held no professional credentials. These two professionals often found themselves in some degree of conflict with their manager and frequently questioned the manager's direction. A direct reporting relationship between a nonmanagerial technical specialist and a generalist manager is often marked by many disputes concerning managerial judgments, and may also be marked by strong territorialism on the part of the professional.

Automatic management credibility is likely to be greatest when the manager is a professional of obviously "higher" standing than the employee. At the other extreme, management credibility is most strained when the manager's standing is rejected by the professional as being nonprofessional.

LEADERSHIP AND THE PROFESSIONAL

A Range of Styles

Much of this book is about leadership, especially in terms of how to form an appropriate leadership style relative to managing the professional employee. *Leadership style* may be described simply as that pattern of behavior exhibited by the leader in working with the group members. Leadership styles may run the gamut from completely closed to thoroughly open.[1] At the closed-end of the scale are the autocratic leaders, those who rule by order and edict. The harshest style is that of the *exploitative autocrat,* a leader who literally exploits the followers in the service of self-interest. One major move along the scale takes us next to the style of the *benevolent autocrat.* The benevolent autocrat also rules by order and edict, but it is a paternalistic rule that is supposedly for the good of all. For many years the paternalism of the benevolent autocrat was evident in the attitudes projected by much of America's business and industrial leadership toward employees: do exactly as you are told without question and you will be well cared for.

Approaching the middle of the scale of leadership styles one encounters the *bureaucratic* style. In many ways fully as onerous as the autocratic styles, the bureaucratic style ordinarily subordinates human considerations to the service of the system. Bureaucratic leadership first and foremost requires rules and procedures for all contingencies and usually places "the book" (as in doing things "by the book") in a position of importance over people. The need for proscriptions of behavior can be so strong that when there is an occurrence or need that is not covered by existing forms and processes, the system can come to a near halt while the leaders struggle with the unknown. The bureaucracy primarily serves the system itself rather than the system's operators or customers.

Continuing toward the open end of the leadership scale one next encounters the *consultative* style of leadership. Under this approach employees are usually given the opportunity to provide their thoughts, feelings, ideas, and suggestions, but the ground rules are such that the leader owes no obligation to utilize anything the employees provide. The guiding philosophy of management operating in a consultative mode is "the buck stops here." Management may routinely ask for input while yet reserving the right to make all decisions at all times regardless of what the employee contributes.

Consultative leadership often exists when management claims to practice true *participative* leadership, the style at the extreme open end of the scale. Many managers who continue to believe they approach management with an honest belief in employee participation are far more consultative in their approach: They ask for input, then incorporate only that which is consistent with their pre-existing beliefs. This in fact represents the greatest shortcoming of participative leadership (the inclusion of all group members in decision-making processes such that all members own a piece of each decision): the ease with which managers, most of whom grew into their positions under partially authoritarian role models, can unconsciously hinder participative processes such that they become consultative and at times even manipulative.

The higher the professional level of a work group, the more the manager will find it necessary to move toward the open end of the scale of leadership styles to accomplish the work of the department. Given the nature of professional work and the advanced state of most professionals' education, the typical professional will not stand still for long under authoritarian leadership. It behooves the manager to examine some fundamental assumptions about human behavior, to get beyond mere verbal tribute to "modern" management, and to assume some of the risks inherent in open leadership styles.

Some Assumptions About People

Douglas McGregor, in his work "The Human Side of Enterprise," wrote of two opposing approaches to management: Theory X and Theory Y.[2] Theory X in its pure state is autocratic leadership. Pure Theory Y is genuine participative leadership. Each of these management theories is based on a number of assumptions; only the first assumption, relating to management in general, is common to both X and Y. That common assumption, valid in any case, is that management remains responsible for organizing all of the elements of productive activity: that is, bringing together the money, people, equipment, and supplies needed to accomplish the organization's goals. Beyond this assumption, however, the two theories proceed in opposite directions. Theory X assumes the following:

- People must be actively managed. They must be directed and motivated, and their actions must be controlled and their behavior modified to fit the needs of the organization. Without this active intervention by management, people would be passive and even resistant to organizational needs. Therefore, people must be persuaded, controlled, rewarded, or punished as necessary to accomplish the aims of the organization.

- The average person is by nature indolent, working as little as possible. The average person lacks ambition, shuns responsibility, and in general prefers to be led.

- The average person is inherently self-centered, resistant to change, and indifferent to the needs of the organization.

Theory Y, on the other hand, is founded upon the following assumptions:

- People are not naturally passive or resistant to organizational needs. If they appear to have become so, this condition is the result of experience in organizations.

- Motivation, development potential, willingness to assume responsibility, and readiness to work toward organizational goals are present in most people. It is management's responsibility to enable people to recognize and develop these characteristics for themselves.

- The essential task of management is to arrange organizational conditions and methods of operation so people can best achieve their own goals by directing their efforts toward the goals of the organization.

Style and Circumstances

Professional or otherwise, not every employee responds in the same way to the same leadership style. However, because the typical professional is generally more receptive to open styles—approaches consistent with Theory Y—it is in the manager's best interest to begin a manager–employee relationship with reliance on an open style. A manager's style may depend largely on individual circumstances, but in starting the relationship with an employee one should initially extend every benefit of the doubt regarding the employee's motivations.

The autocratic leader simply operates under Theory X assumptions, choosing to make all the decisions and handing them down as orders and instructions. The participative leader generally ascribes to Theory Y assumptions and encourages employees to participate in joint processes.

The manager has a choice of leadership styles ranging from extremely closed to extremely open. The trick is to know when any particular style or approach is appropriate. There may be some Theory X people in the department (those few who actually prefer to be led and have their thinking done for them), but they are likely to be a minority. However, there may also be a number of Theory Y people who are self-motivated and capable of significant self-direction. This should be especially true in departments employing large numbers of professionals. Although the same rules (personnel policies) apply uniformly to all employees, the manager deals differently with individuals in other ways. For some, the manager consults and invites their participation; for others the manager simply directs.

Theories aside, a manager must avoid making assumptions about people. Rather, it is necessary to know the employees and to try to understand each one both as a person and a producer. By working with people over a period of time, and especially by working at the business of getting to know them, one can learn a great deal about each individual's likes, dislikes, and capabilities. It is essential to learn about the people as individuals and then lead accordingly. If a certain employee genuinely prefers orders and instructions, and this attitude is not consistent with job requirements, then use orders and instructions. Although many health care workers seem to prefer participative leadership, not everyone desires this same consideration. Sufficient flexibility must be maintained to accommodate the employee who wants or requires authoritarian supervision. It is fully as unfair to expect people to become what they do not want to be as it is to allow a rigid structure to stifle those other employees who feel they have something to contribute.

No single style of leadership is appropriate to all people and all situations at all times. There is now more reason than ever to believe that consultative and participative leadership is most appropriate to modern health care organizations and today's educated workers.

Much can be said about what leadership is and is not, but when all is said and done one finds that only a single factor truly characterizes, or "defines," a leader: the acceptance of the followers.[3] For this critical factor to be present in the relationship developed between the manager and the professional employee, the professional must

- respect the manager's technical knowledge;
- accept the manager's organizational authority and respect the manager's skill in using that authority; and
- respect the manager's ability to blend the technical and managerial sides of the management role fairly and justly.

The manager accrues little, if any, acceptance by virtue of organizational authority. Most of what the manager acquires in the way of willing acceptance must be earned. It can thus be suggested that to lead the professional employee successfully, the manager must provide a broad framework for employee action, provide the employee with every opportunity to be self-led, and impose specific direction only after all else has failed and the employee has demonstrated the need to be taken by the hand.

DELEGATION: THE SAME, BUT DIFFERENT

How Well Do You Delegate?

Most managers believe in the necessity of delegation. Most are certainly capable of paying verbal tribute to delegation and its value and, if questioned, most would convey the belief that they delegate reasonably well. However, a great many managers who think that they delegate reasonably well—or who think consciously of delegation little if at all, considering it as no more than simply handing out work—actually delegate poorly and incompletely. Far too many managers simply assign work to a person without paying sufficient attention to how the person is prepared and why the process is used at all.

Many managers fall into a classic time trap regarding delegation. During times of normal or seemingly reasonable activity, the possibility of delegation of work to subordinates simply does not occur to them. Rather, thoughts like "I really need to delegate some of this to get relief from some of this overload" usually arise only when the load is heaviest and time is tightest. These thoughts are invariably followed at once by thoughts such as, "But it will take time to show someone how to do it—time I don't have at present."

Ordinarily the manager concedes to the pressure of time and takes care of the task in question personally. Perhaps the manager also mentally promises to delegate this to someone "after the rush is over." However, when the urgency dissipates, the thoughts of delegation fade as well. The manager gives no more thought to the need for delegation until that need is again brought to the fore by the constraints of the time trap.

It is essential for the manager to realize that the time savings of delegation are rarely if ever immediate. One must accept the need to spend more time now—even when time is tightest and the backlog of work is greatest—to assure time savings that will come weeks or even months in the future.

Obligation to Delegate

The manager has a fundamental obligation to him- or herself and to the employees to practice proper delegation. The manager's basic charge is to get things done *through people*, and to be able to do so effectively the manager must delegate in order to

- avoid falling into the working trap, spending most of the time on technical task work and simply serving primarily as one more pair of hands in the department;
- function effectively as a member of the organization's management team (which one cannot do if consumed with nonmanagerial tasks); and
- enhance the possibility of promotion to a position of greater responsibility. (Rarely will an enlightened higher management promote a department manager who has not demonstrated skill at proper delegation.)

Likewise the manager owes the employees a number of considerations that are best served through proper delegation. These include

- the opportunity to learn and grow on the job;
- the opportunity to prove themselves able to handle additional responsibility; and
- the chance to find stimulation, interest, and challenge in their work.

The Delegation Process

The customary delegation pattern consists of four significant phases:

1. *Select and organize the task.* The task selected for delegation should be one that the manager should not have to do. That is, it must be technical and not managerial in nature. Pure managerial tasks—making planning and budgeting decisions, making policy decisions, handling personnel problems or other matters of personnel administration (hiring, firing, promotional decisions, and so on)—cannot be delegated. The

task selected for delegation should be a nonmanagerial task that is expected to recur at least often enough to make the time and effort of delegation worthwhile.

2. *Select the appropriate person.* The process of selecting an employee to whom to delegate a given task is admittedly a judgmental process which the manager learns through experience. From the perspective of the manager, the employee selected should

   - be ready to assume some additional responsibility;
   - have regular assignments well under control;
   - be neither obviously overqualified nor underqualified for the task; and
   - appear to possess capabilities that could be put to productive use on this particular task.

3. *Instruct and motivate the person.* Delegation is far more than handing a task to an employee and expecting that it will be done. The manager must be able to provide the employee with

   - the reason for the task: why it is important that this must be done;
   - sufficient authority to accomplish the expected results;
   - thorough instructions, provided at the employee's level of language and understanding;
   - understanding of what's in it for the employee (a chance to learn, to add variety to the work, to become more versatile and potentially more valuable, and so on); and
   - a clear understanding of what results are expected and when they are to be delivered.

4. *Maintain reasonable control.* It is not enough to assure that the employee is well launched on the task; it is also necessary to assure that he or she remains on course. Control of delegation is largely a matter of communication between manager and employee. The frequency and intensity of this communication depend significantly on the manager's assessment of the employee. One must know the employees well enough to be able to judge who needs what degree of control or assistance. The employees in a group are bound to differ from each other in a number of ways. Some must be checked frequently and monitored closely; some may be allowed to operate almost completely independently. However, regardless of how much or how little guidance a par-

ticular employee requires, the manager should avoid solving the employee's problems for him or her and focus instead on teaching employees how to solve their own problems.

The Professional: Some Important Differences

The foregoing phases of delegation can be expanded to some extent for the manager of professional employees. The processes remain essentially the same; however, in some instances the emphasis is different.

- Under the first phase ("select and organize the task"), strong emphasis should be placed on defining the results required of task completion. The task must of course be a technical (i.e., a nonmanagerial) task, but in organizing the task the manager may pay less attention to defining method and more attention to defining results.

- Everything noted under the second phase ("select the appropriate person"), applies to the professional employee. Professional or nonprofessional, the employee to whom a task is delegated must be appropriately matched to the task according to qualifications, and must be ready and able to take on the new assignment.

- Under the third phase ("instruct and motivate the person"), the motivational aspects of delegation certainly remain the same. Instruction, however, should be different in the same sense that the second phase is different for the professional: Rather than dwell on method or procedure, instruction should focus on conveying clear understanding of expected results and should culminate in mutual agreement on those expected results.

- The human considerations in the fourth phase ("maintain reasonable control") remain essentially the same: relative closeness of control depends on the manager's assessment of the employee, professional or not. There are, however, some likely differences in focus. In following up with the professional, the manager is more likely able to focus on actual progress and less on adherence to procedure. The manager should be able to expect the professional's tendency toward operating autonomy to come through and should indeed be hesitant to provide handholding guidance. This is not to say that close control is not necessary from time to time, but is simply to suggest that the professional should be given reasonable latitude unless (or until) the employee has proven the need for close supervision. (The professional employee who has proven the need for close supervision presents the manager with a challenge that extends well beyond delegation.)

The key to the process of delegating to the professional employee is the complete mutual understanding of and agreement with the results expected of the employee. The employee's methods for achieving those results may be flexible, and generally up to the employee, as long as they fall within the realm of what is legal, moral, and ethical, and within the bounds of accepted practice.

Authority and Responsibility

It is authority—specifically, task performance authority—that one delegates, not responsibility. The distinction is an important one. When delegating, the manager gives over a certain amount of task performance authority to a subordinate. The manager actually sheds—willingly gives up—this task performance authority and can again perform the task that was delegated away only by recalling that authority. One can think of the manager's total authority as a divisible physical object such as a pie; in delegation, the manager removes a slice of this authority and assigns it to a subordinate. This slice of authority now belongs to the employee.

Responsibility, however, is an entirely different matter. The responsibility for the outcome of the task cannot be shed. Rather, the responsibility is replicated at an additional level; the manager holds the employee responsible for task performance, but the manager remains responsible to higher authority as if still performing the task personally.

It is perhaps the relationship between authority and responsibility that leaves many managers uncomfortable with delegation. They know—or at least sense, if they do not consciously think such thoughts—that they remain responsible for the outcomes produced by others. This discomfort probably has a lot to do with encouraging some managers to behave as though acting out the old saying, *If you want something done right, do it yourself.*

However, the manager cannot do everything alone. Thus the necessity of delegation, to enable the manager to fulfill the essential function of getting things done through people. One's discomfort with carrying full responsibility should provide the manager with all the motivation necessary to focus on thorough, effective delegation, and thus on the development of subordinates who will perform responsibly.

The Habit of Delegation

Proper delegation is a habit as surely as sloppy, halfway delegation is a habit. Proper delegation is simple to absorb in concept: the steps are few and mostly common sense. The truly difficult part is breaking old habits and replacing them with new, healthier habits. To do so, one must begin by delegating one or two simple tasks and then analyzing their cycle, from delegation (including instruction), through follow-up, in painstaking detail, perhaps even following written checklists and writing notes to ones self on a daily basis. This must be done repeatedly until the thoroughness of attention to the process literally becomes automatic. Once the process is part of the manager's behavior pattern—once it is *truly* a habit—proper delegation pays dividends for the remainder of one's management career.

THE PROFESSIONAL AND CHANGE

No single group or classification of employees has a monopoly on resistance to change. Rigidity and inflexibility may be found at all levels of the organization. However, one might expect the professional employee to be on average generally more amenable to change because of the professional's advanced education and broader perspective. But as many managers have discovered, the professional employee may be as fully resistant to change as any other employee. It depends entirely on how the employee is approached and how the particular change is presented.

Basis for Resistance

As far as the majority of people are concerned, change is threatening. Change threatens one's security by altering the environment, and change disturbs one's equilibrium, the state of balance most persons automatically seek to maintain with their surroundings at all times.

Most persons do indeed seek a degree of comfort relative to their surroundings, and they continually make adjustments intended to preserve their equilibrium. Because change—especially unwanted or unheralded change—threatens to disturb one's equilibrium, it becomes a threat to one's sense of security. As a result, one reacts in completely human fashion by attempting to counter the threat by resisting the change.

In work organizations, resistance to change is brought about primarily by

- organizational changes, in which the reporting relationships of managers and departments are altered;
- management changes, in which one must henceforth report to a new superior;
- changes in work methods and procedures, and in the policies of the organization;

- job restructuring, in which task responsibilities area added or taken away; and
- the introduction of new technology and new equipment.

It is primarily the unknown that fosters resistance or intensifies what otherwise might be only nominal resistance. In short, any item in the foregoing list can generate resistance even if approached with full knowledge and plenty of warning. If it comes on the employee by surprise, though, then intense resistance is practically assured. When a change is not a surprise, when it is approached with the full knowledge of everyone involved, much of the unknown becomes known and the chances of success are greatly increased.

The Manager's Approach

When approaching employees with change a manager can

- *Tell* them what to do. This is simply giving orders: "Here it is, folks—do it this way starting now." This way is quick and straight to the point. However, it is also the way to generate maximum resistance because it presents a major threat to the employees and it suggests the manager expects them to blindly obey. The telling route is rarely appropriate and should be reserved as a last resort, used only after the reasons for the change are fully revealed to the employees.
- *Convince* them of what must be done. This approach at least can be used with most employees. Many changes, especially in health care, are required by regulations and mandates that are well beyond the control of the individual manager. One may not be convinced of the value of a given change, or of the reasoning behind it, but may nevertheless be convinced that the change must indeed be made. And the employee who understands why a change is unavoidable is less likely to be resistant.
- *Involve* them in assessing the need for change and in determining the form and substance of the change. This may not always be possible (for instance, where changes mandated by external regulatory agencies are concerned), and it may not always be practical because of time constraints. However, much of the time there is ample opportunity to involve the employees legitimately.

Employee Involvement in Addressing Change

Employee involvement in the management of change is important for a number of reasons, significant among which are the following:

- Involvement requires time. The time it takes to introduce the possible need for change and determine how to act eliminates the element of surprise and minimizes the impact of the unknown.

- Having contributed to the form and substance of a change, employees are more likely to be accepting of it because they own a piece of the change.

- The employees—those people who do the hands-on work day in and day out—possess detailed information about the performance of the work. Managers, systems analysts, consultants, and the like may have more appropriate perspectives on overall processes and how they fit together, but as far as specific tasks are concerned nobody knows the intimate details better than the people who do the work every day. This is a source of knowledge that the manager should always seek to tap.

The nature of professional work also holds implications for the management of change. Because much of the focus in dealing with the professional is on expected results, the manager should concentrate on employee involvement that emphasizes the determination of and agreement on expected results. As much as possible of the concern for specific methods—how the desired results are obtained—should be left to the discretion and judgment of the professional employee.

To enjoy the greatest chance of successfully managing change, the manager should

- *inform* employees as early as possible of what is likely to happen;

- *plan* thoroughly;

- *communicate* fully;

- *convince* employees as necessary;

- *involve* employees whenever the circumstances of the change permit; and

- *monitor* implementation to ensure that decisions are adjusted and plans are fine-tuned as necessary.

The manager should consider the department's professional employees to be the principal players in implementing change. Knowledge and involvement are the keys to success, and the employee who knows what is happening and is involved in making it happen is less likely to resist. Employees resist most strongly when a change appears to be driven by outside forces, coming completely and uncontrollably from outside themselves. The manager eventually discovers that it is not *change* that is resisted nearly as much as *being changed.*

METHODS IMPROVEMENT

Every worker has a potentially valuable role to play in improving the methods by which the work is accomplished. As noted, nobody knows the inner working details of a job better than the person who does it every day. This detailed knowledge is essential in methods improvement; precisely how a task is performed is the necessary starting point in working to improve the performance of that task.

The professional employee is especially important in the improvement of methods because

- the professional's breadth of knowledge in the field, both theoretical and practical, is a source of a variety of work-improvement options; and

- the creative nature of much professional work suggests that the professional knows not just what to do but also how to determine what to do.

The professional employee often makes an effective key person in a methods improvement undertaking, such as chairing a quality circle or leading a work simplification team. In all probability the professional knows the work far better than the manager does. The manager, even though probably a professional as well, has necessarily been growing away from the technical work in some respects while growing as a manager. To succeed in improving the methods by which the work is accomplished, the manager must regard the department's professionals as the most potentially valuable source of improvement knowledge.

EMPLOYEE PROBLEMS

Occasionally managers tend to treat their professional employees much like parents often treat the oldest child in the family: "You are more advanced, so we can expect more of you." (Or, using another form of the same basic message, "You're older—you should know better.")

The you-should-know-better attitude is fine as long as it is expressed properly and is not carried to extremes as far as the technical work of the profession is concerned. However, this attitude is not generally appropriate regarding adherence to the policies and work rules of the organization.

In applying rules and policies, consistency must be observed in dealings with all employees. The professional employee should not be held to more rigid standards of behavior simply because of being a professional ("You should know better"). On the other hand, neither should the professional be allowed to get away with more simply because of his or her professional status. Rather, policies and work rules must be applied equally to all employees regardless of qualifications or classification, and the manager must take pains to ensure that everyone receives equal treatment.

The professional is fully as human and unpredictable as any other employee when it comes to the likelihood of personal problems, variations in personality, and behavior that might give rise to employee problems. A manager's long-run experience will show that professional employees can at times be fully as great a source of discipline and behavior problems as can be nonprofessional employees. When the kinds of problems presented by employees are considered, one often finds that the problems presented by professionals are more complex and difficult to deal with than the problems presented by their nonprofessional colleagues. Especially troublesome is the occasional professional who takes advantage of professional status to demand professional treatment, without extending the appropriate behavior in return (refer to Chapter 5).

COMMUNICATION AND THE PROFESSIONAL

The Professional and the "Inside" Language

It would be pertinent to repeat for the manager of professionals all the good advice that can be offered for communication as it applies to the manager of any employees, professional or otherwise. This discussion, however, is limited to those aspects of communication in which professional status or professionalism make a difference.

Each function within the modern health care organization includes some amount of what may be referred to as "inside language"—the specialized jargon that is unique to that particular occupation or profession. Those who work in building services or maintenance have special terms that they use regularly, a few of which might be unfamiliar to persons who work in other departments, and completely foreign to persons outside of health care. Similarly, food service workers use a few terms that have meaning to only them. Physicians, dentists, and pharmacists most certainly have inside languages that have evolved within their respective disciplines.

Development of "Inside" Language

Inside languages are an inevitable outgrowth of the development of any area of concentrated specialized activity. The more concentrated the specialty and, in the case of the health professions, the higher on the professional scale an occupation resides, the more extensive this inside language is and the more incomprehensible it is to outsiders.

Inside languages develop for perfectly logical reasons. As advances are made in any aspect of life or any area of business activity, the need arises for describing concepts, conditions, problems, and even physical objects in a way that clearly identifies these within the context of the growing specialty as different from anything else in the world.

The needed words come from two sources: existing words that are given new meanings for specific purposes and new words coined to represent that which did not previously exist. As a simple example, consider the effect the advent of the internal combustion engine, and specifically the automobile, had on the English language during the early half of the twentieth century. The invention of the automobile gave us terms such as *overdrive, carburetor, spark plug, headlight,* and *crankshaft* that may not have previously existed or that resulted from the combination of existing words in a new context. The automobile also gave new meaning to old words in the language, such as *bumper, starter, distributor, clutch,* and *differential.* In similar fashion, every bit of advancing technology has expanded the language. And every profession that has emerged and evolved has built its special language along the way.

Clearly our basic language must be dynamic; it must be able to shift and expand as our knowledge increases. It is thus fully understandable that an inside language should develop within any activity. It serves a clear purpose in describing, in terms as specific as possible, what goes on within that activity. Some may also say, however, in perhaps less-than-kindly fashion, that the purpose of an inside language is to elevate the specialty and define it as a closed club of sorts. Though probably not an expressed purpose of an inside language, this is undoubtedly an effect of such a language. An inside language certainly heightens the mystique surrounding any given occupation, and in addition serves to define the territory about that occupation. Relative to territory, the presence of the inside language says that one must not enter unless qualified. Command of the inside language is a qualification, admittedly superficial, but certainly highly visible, for entry into someone's territory. In short, if you don't speak the language, don't bother to knock.

Nurses have a language of their own, and human resources practitioners have a language of their own. Laboratory employees, radiology employees, physical therapists, psychologists, social workers, occupational therapists, physicians, and many others have their own inside languages. Fortunately, many of these inside languages have some terms in common so they are not entirely different from each other. For example, some of the nurses' inside language is the same as part of the physicians' inside language, and it is largely these areas of overlap that provide the interprofessional points of contact through which much communication flows. Occasionally, however, there emerges an inside language that has few, if any, points of overlap with other inside languages.

Computerese: In a World of Its Own

A glaring example of a highly restrictive inside language is found in the field of computers and electronic information processing and management. This specialty area is filled with terms, and abbreviations, and acronyms that are used freely in normal interchange, often without sufficient explanation. One hears about RAM, ROM, and CPU often without being told they mean *random-access memory, read-only memory,* and *central processing unit.* Many times the full terms are used without further explanation, so people who are not literate in computer language have no understanding of the concepts represented. Old, otherwise familiar words are used in new combinations and with entirely new meaning, such as *mainframe, terminal, disk, peripheral, online,* and *real time.* Inside language is extremely concentrated in information management, with few areas of overlap with the languages of other specialties. Computers and information management seem so incomprehensible to many people because of the language: computerese is essentially a language in its own right, and the necessity to confront this language to become computer literate may well be a strong factor in perpetuating "computer phobia" in some people.

Using the Professional's Language

One of the major problems commonly encountered in communication involving professionals is the disregard for the need to structure any given communication to suit the needs and capabilities of the audience. In communicating, the professional

- may freely use inside language when communicating with other professionals in the same specialty;
- must use a lesser level of special terminology when relating to persons outside the specific specialty, but still within the same industry (health care); and
- must use a third and general level of language when relating to persons outside of both the specific specialty and the industry.

The manager has a key role to fulfill in professional communication. It is all too easy for the manager to perpetuate foggy communication by simply joining in with some professionals in the group and relying on restrictive inside language in all contacts. This is not unusual when the manager has risen through the ranks in the same profession. Rather, it should fall to the manager to serve constantly as a facilitator and, as necessary, a translator in communication between the professional group and others. This role should extend to instruction and guidance in how to structure reports, memoranda, and other documents to the needs of a specific audience, and how to do likewise for the audiences that must listen to professionals' oral presentations.

Some professionals tend to use language to make themselves appear knowledgeable and important, to elevate the mystique of the profession, and to isolate and protect the profession's territory. However, the primary purpose of language should be to communicate; that is, to transfer meaning. As the primary source of worker guidance and the department's major point of contact with the rest of the organization, the manager has a strong interest in ensuring that the department's contributions are presented such that they are completely understood by those who need to know.

AN OPEN-ENDED TASK

On any given day the professional employee can present the manager with any problem or challenge that can be brought by the nonprofessional—and then some. Any advice that may apply to the management of anyone can apply to the management of the professional; additional requirements on the manager call for the constant awareness of the sometimes subtle, and sometimes glaring, differences presented by the professional employee. In addition to the normal requirements of managing any employee, in the day-to-day management of the health care professional the manager must

- help the professional employee identify and pursue objectives that are consistent with the objectives of the department and the organization;

- work to ensure consistency between the priorities of the employee's profession and the priorities of the department and the organization;

- strive to establish and maintain management credibility in a clear leadership role relative to the individual professional employee; and

- establish and maintain a working communication link between the individual professional and all other employees.

NOTES

1. C. R. McConnell, *The Effective Health Care Supervisor, Fifth Edition* (Gaithersburg, MD: Aspen Publishers, Inc., 2002), 150–152.

2. D. M. McGregor, The Human Side of Enterprise, *Management Review* 46, no. 11 (November 1957): 22–28; 88–92.
3. C. R. McConnell, *The Effective Health Care Supervisor, Fifth Edition*, pp. 154–155.

QUESTIONS AND ACTIVITIES

1. Explain in detail why the high-skill professional can sometimes be more difficult to manage than other employees.

2. If the manager is of "lower" professional status than some of the employees, how might the manager compensate for this difference in managing professional employees?

3. From the perspective of a department manager, explain the fallacy inherent in the statement: If you want something done right, do it yourself.

4. Describe a work group in which the manager probably has to exercise a variety of leadership styles, and explain why this variety of styles might be necessary.

5. Explain why so much emphasis is placed on focusing on expected results in managing the professional employee.

6. Using at least two examples, describe how some professionals might sometimes be called upon to function as team players and sometimes be expected to function as lone operators.

7. Given that most managers agree on the importance of delegation, explain why so many managers fail to delegate properly.

8. Provide one example of an occupation that has its own "inside language. Describe the circumstances under which this language might be used either partially or in full and when it should be completely avoided.

9. Fully explain why employee retention can be an important consideration even at times when replacement employees are readily available.

10. Describe the problems that are likely to ensue if the professional employee does not respect the level of the department manager's technical knowledge.

11. Describe how you might recommend proceeding with the professional employee who has proven through behavior that he or she requires close supervision.

QUESTIONS AND ACTIVITIES *(continued)*

12. Describe the potential negative effects of territorialism among groups of professional employees within an organization.

13. Explain why some employees seem to "want or require authoritarian supervision."

14. Fully explain why the motivation of the employee to perform is usually central to successful delegation.

15. During times when certain skills are in short supply, health care organizations have been known to attempt luring employees from each other with improved salaries and benefits. What are the potential effects of this practice?

16. Describe the circumstances when the department manager should take care of unanticipated nonmanagerial tasks personally rather than delegate them to employees.

17. A department has just suddenly and inexplicably lost its manager, and the employees have been told that a new manager will soon arrive. Although the former manager was feared by some and disliked by many, most staff members demonstrate some uneasiness about getting a new manager. Explain why the uneasiness exists.

18. Explain why many managers who claim to be participative, and believe they are participative, are actually consultative in style.

19. Provide several examples of functions that the manager cannot delegate and explain why these functions cannot be delegated.

20. Describe the elements of a supply-and-demand cycle for an occupation (such as registered nurse). Suggestion: Consider the likely effects of the employment market on what is in the supply "pipeline" (mainly schools) at any given time.

CHAPTER 10

The Professional as a Manager

The right of commanding is no longer an advantage transmitted by nature;
like an inheritance, it is the fruit of labors, the price of courage.

—Voltaire

This Chapter Will:

► Examine the dual role—technical specialist and management generalist—of the professional who is employed as a manager, and consider when the halves of this role are out of balance;

► Explore some special problems and barriers to effectiveness frequently encountered by professional employees who enter management;

► Confirm the legitimacy of management, which may necessarily become a second career for many professionals, as a profession in its own right, and suggest the need for equal dedication to parallel careers; and

► Review the changes occurring in the role of the health care department manager because of reengineering, downsizing, organizational flattening, and mergers and other affiliations.

TWO HATS: SPECIALIST AND MANAGER

Assuming the Parallel Career

The professional who is asked to assume a managerial position is being asked to take on a second occupation to an extent that amounts to pursuing a second and parallel career. Management positions turn over as other positions do, and vacant management positions are often filled from the ranks of the work group. There are both advantages and disadvantages to having a particular member of a work group step up to the position of group leader; on occasion, for any of several reasons, the new manager of the group may come from outside of the organization.

Although familiarity with the specific organizational setting may be helpful to the new manager, such familiarity is certainly not a requirement of a group's new manager. However, there is one firm requirement of the individual who is to assume command of any work group: In addition to possessing (one would hope) some management skill, the individual must be intimately knowledgeable of the kinds of work that the group performs. Because many work groups within the health care institution include professional employees, and because the manager's technical qualifications must essentially be equivalent to the qualifications found in the department, the career ladder of a professional may logically be extended to include the management of that specialty.

The professional who enters management must exist forever after in a two-hat situation. This person must wear the hat of the professional, that is, the technical specialist, and render judgment on countless technical matters concerning the profession. But this person must also wear the hat of the manager, and effect the application of techniques that are generic in nature, processes that apply horizontally across the organization regardless of the nature of one's individual specialty. The professional in a management role must be both specialist and generalist. As a professional, the person is trained as a specialist in a particular field. As a manager, however, it remains largely up to the individual to recognize the need to become a generalist and to seek out independently sources of education and assistance.

The average employee who progresses from the ranks into management is usually well grounded in a working specialty. In this sense all employees, professionals and nonprofessionals alike, are functional specialists. For instance, the person who works for several years in the housekeeping department and who has performed a number of housekeeping tasks and become a specialist in the work of the department brings all of this experience into supervision when promoted. At the very least the nonprofessional is a specialist by way of experience.

The professional employee is usually a specialist by virtue of experience. However, experience is only part of a professional's qualifications as a specialist: the remaining criteria defining the professional as a specialist are education and accreditation. The professional entering management brings both credentials and experience to the job. In this regard the person is usually eminently qualified to wear the manager's technical hat. However, the individual may not be nearly as qualified to wear the managerial hat.

Examples of Professional Managers

Many persons put a great deal of time, money, and effort into becoming professionals. It is only after acquiring a prescribed amount of education and perhaps acquiring the appropriate accreditation that an individual can legitimately lay claim to professional status. Consider the following cases of individuals who are representative of many persons working in health care organizations:

- Kathleen J. completed a three-year diploma program and passed a state licensing examination before she could use the designation of registered nurse (R.N.).

- Arthur W. spent four years at a university earning a technical degree and the right to use the title of biomedical engineer.

- Janice R. went through a two-year hospital-based program consisting of both classroom work and clinical experience before she could become licensed as a radiology technician.

- William P. completed four years of college to become an accountant. After several required years of work experience he passed an examination and earned the right to use the designation of certified public accountant (C.P.A.).

- Maureen L. had to complete a four-year college program and acquire professional registry to earn the designation of registered record administrator (R.R.A.).

In considering the foregoing, note the amount of work implied in the process of attaining professional status and note as well the length of time devoted by each person. Becoming a professional is at times a difficult and time-consuming process, stretching as long as six, seven, or even eight years for some of the high-skill professionals. Imagine that each of the persons mentioned has been promoted to a management position, and consider how much preparation each may have been afforded.

- Kathleen, the registered nurse, had only a few hours of management orientation in the form of a single supervisory skills seminar. She had been exposed to a great deal of continuing education through nursing inservice education, but all of this was clinical in nature.

- Arthur, the biomedical engineer, had absolutely no orientation or other preparation relating to management.

- Janice, the radiology technician, was sent to a two-day management program the month after she was promoted to the position of supervising technician.

- William, the accountant, had perhaps four college courses—less than 10 percent of his undergraduate education—that could be described as management courses. However, they were largely concerned with management theory, organization theory, and long-range planning and other matters that are primarily the concern of top management.

- Maureen, the record administrator, had several courses in the college program intended to orient her toward the management of a health care institution's record department. However, none of this management education was concerned with how to handle day-to-day operating problems, or how to deal with a supervisor's area of greatest concern: people problems.

Well Trained and Untrained

The professional who enters management is often extremely well trained in the specialty but trained minimally, or not at all, in matters of management. Persons become professionals by seeking out the appropriate programs, gaining entry, and working toward professional qualifications. However, these same people become managers by virtue of organizational edict; that is, they are simply appointed. Precisely at this stage some employees and organizations commit a classic error—assuming that because people have been appointed and given appropriate titles, they are suddenly managers in the true sense of the word. However, organizational edict does not automatically make a manager of someone who is not adequately trained or appropriately oriented to management any more than the mere conferral of the appropriate title could turn an untrained person into a nurse, an accountant, a biomedical engineer, or any other professional.

The professional entering management, then, is usually well trained at wearing the hat of the specialist and trained little, or not at all, in wearing the hat of a manager. Although each side of the role is equally important, and even though one side or the other will necessarily dominate at times, many such persons exhibit a long-run tendency that is fully understandable under the circumstances: they tend to favor wearing the hat that fits best, leaning toward the one of their two roles in which they find themselves more comfortable.

Manager's Complaints

Listen to some of the common complaints of certain managers. It is possible, by identifying those aspects of the job that lie at the heart of these complaints, to identify those persons on whom the management hat does not fit especially comfortably. The following illustrations reveal some indications of ill-fitting management hats:

- "Good grief, budget time again? Why does it always happen this way? I need to get some real work done, but I wind up pushing numbers around instead. And what for? It's just a game. I pad the figures because I know that somebody is going to cut them. Somebody cuts the figures because they assume I padded them, so we go 'round and 'round until we've wasted a lot of time and I come out of it with less money than I really need to run the department. It's such a disruptive process, and anyway the numbers are all Greek to me."

- "Yes, I know I'm late with my performance appraisals. It's just that things have really been popping and the census has been up for weeks and there have been all sorts of things to be done. Anyway I guess these found their way to the bottom of the basket and I forgot about them. Or I just put them off a few times before I *really* forgot about them. Anyway I hate to get all wrapped up in these. They're so frustrating to write up, and I'm always uncomfortable talking them out with employees. For all the time these appraisals take—we do them because the human resources department makes us do them, you know—I really don't see what good they accomplish."

- "It's the nagging little problems—the stuff that comes up every day, like employees squabbling, someone complaining or objecting to an assignment, people calling in sick and causing me to juggle the schedule—that really bugs me. I could get some real work done around here if it weren't for all these nagging little problems that keep popping up."

- "Listen, gang, I know I'm supposed to be the boss of this outfit, but don't forget that my background is the same as yours and I'm a lot more like you than like those people in top management. I know that you don't like this latest change in policy. Well, I don't like it any more than you do—but they made me do it."

- "Well, yes, I know that I should have given her a warning two months ago and maybe even one before that when the problem first came up. But I didn't because, well, do you know how difficult it really is to discipline someone you've known and liked for years?"

- "Leave of absence policy? Sure, we've got one in the personnel policy manual. Right there—the fattest book on the shelf. Talk about a paper mill! No, I don't know especially what it says but you can take the book and dig it out for yourself."

- "Do you believe it—now I'm not supposed to deal with sales representatives directly. I'm expected to see that all the reps go through the purchasing department. Talk about adding unnecessary steps and building a bureaucracy!"

- "The way things are going, before long I'm going to be running the whole operation by myself. I'm already putting in more than 10 hours a day and the pile is still growing."

- "If I haven't learned anything else on this job, I've certainly learned that if you want something done right you had better do it yourself."

The list could go on at considerably greater length, but the foundation of the current point has been adequately established. The manager is feeling the pinch of the management hat, reacting out of frustration and insecurity and taking refuge under the technical hat. Those processes that can be described as generic to management because they apply organizationally across the board—such as budgeting and performance appraisal—appear as somewhat mysterious, not completely understood activities that come to be regarded as elements of interference rather than the vital elements of management that they are. The disciplinary problems, other people problems, and in general all those "nagging little problems" are likewise seen as annoyances rather than legitimate obstacles to be overcome in the process of getting things done through people. What is seen as real work is the work of the technical specialty. Overlooked is the reality that the true task of the manager is largely to serve as a facilitator in the process of getting the real work done by the employees.

The manager's reaction embodied in, "Don't blame me—they made me do it" illustrates an unwillingness to identify with management and lend support to instructions or to policy changes that may not meet with favor in the work group. To espouse such a position is to deny one's responsibility for supporting the objectives of the organization by taking an approach that says, in effect, "I'm only one of the troops, just like you are—so please don't dislike me," rather than pursuing the more difficult and personally riskier course of attempting to gain acceptance through explanation and persuasion.

The manager who complains about the work group, feels it necessary to work 10 hours a day, and believes that if you want something done right you had better do it yourself has paid little attention to some of the most important reasons for the manager's existence. The true manager teaches employees, coaches employees, and delegates to employees. It is sometimes easier—at least in the short run—to take care of many problems and accomplish many tasks by putting in extra hours and assuming the burden oneself. However, many matters so addressed should rightly be considered the province of the technical specialist. The manager is charged with the quite different and admittedly more difficult task of developing employees to the point where they are fully capable of handling those tasks that seem to threaten to turn the manager into a dedicated workaholic.

The Ill-Fitting Management Hat

The signs of the ill-fitting management hat are many. Many managers continually take refuge under the hat of the technical specialist. This is understandable considering the professional employee's degree of familiarity with the occupation, and also considering the professional's unfamiliarity and discomfort with some of the processes of management. However, the simple knowledge of the likely imbalance between the two roles should be sufficient to inspire some managers to improve their capability and performance in the management sphere. Both sides of the manager's role are extremely important. A working knowledge of the technical specialty remains important at most levels in the health care management hierarchy. Particularly in the lower levels of management, the generalist side of the role—that is, the management side—is neither more nor less important than the specialist side. It is simply different.

Although most managers in the health care organization's hierarchy have a need to be both technical specialist and management generalist, there is also a place in the management hierarchy for the pure management generalist. However, the few management generalists in the organization are usually found only in the upper reaches of the hierarchy in positions of multidepartmental responsibility.

In the health care organization, administration is the province of the pure management generalist. Administrators of health institutions come from a variety of backgrounds, with many of them rising out of the management of certain specialties and having perhaps broadened their scope through studies in administration. It matters little whether the institution's administrator may have originally trained as an accountant, a registered nurse, an attorney, or a physician as long as that person made the necessary transition from specialist to generalist while rising toward the top of the organizational pyramid. However, rarely does one encounter the head of a functional specialty who did not begin as a practitioner within that specialty. Rarely does one encounter, for example, a director of nursing service who is not a registered nurse, a medical record manager who was not a medical record practitioner, a director of finance who was not an accountant, or a director of physical therapy who was not a physical therapist.

A CONSTANT BALANCING ACT

Some professionals who take on the management of departments never completely adapt to the dual role of professional and manager, and never develop an appropriate balance between the two sides of the role. Their behavior often sums up their attitude: once a specialist, always a specialist. Such persons tend to give the technical side of the role the majority of their interest and attention, their priority treatment, and certainly their favor. Never having become sufficiently comfortable with the management role to enjoy what they are doing, they take refuge in their strengths and minimize the importance of their weaknesses.

The dedicated professional often has far more difficulty than the nonprofessional in balancing the roles of specialist and manager. The professional has devoted far more time, effort, and commitment to becoming a specialist and has probably done so at least partly because of an attraction or an aptitude for that kind of work. Some may indeed like their work so well that, although they do not necessarily refuse promotion to management, they show an inclination to subordinate the influence of the management side of the role so that it does not intrude too far into the favored territory.

Although the enthusiasm of many professionals for their own fields—that is, they sincerely like what they do—is important, a liking for management is essential for success in management. Often a liking for a given activity is strongly influenced by one's degree of familiarity or level of comfort with the elements of that activity. Quite simply, the more a person knows about a given activity, the more that person is inclined to like that activity. Conversely one may be more readily inclined to dislike an activity that seems bewildering, strange, or discomforting.

It has been suggested that the professional who enters management is faced with the necessity to become grounded in management and get up to speed. Once in management, the individual discovers that to remain effective as a technical professional and as a manager it is necessary to try to remain current in two career fields. Staying current with the latest developments in a technical specialty is a sizable task in itself; getting fully up to speed and remaining current with just those things that have a bearing on one's management role is an unending task, considering the scope and breadth of management. Often one cannot help but let both sides of the role suffer to some extent. However, the technical side is more likely to receive most of the conscientious attention.

The professional employed as a manager has all the problems of any other manager, and also has most of the problems that confront the working professional who is not a manager.

THE EGO BARRIER

Some Are More Special Than Others?

Probably few, if any, health professional do not believe that their professions are of considerable importance to their organizations. This is to be expected; to find any significant measure of fulfillment in work, one would probably have to regard one's occupation as being of significant value to the organization and to its patients. However, the potential for problems exists when an individual professional behaves as though that particular working specialty is more important than other occupations in the organization. If a professional who carries an inflated regard for the importance of a given profession happens to be the manager of a department, the seeds of interdepartmental conflict are present.

Regardless of background or of how one may have entered management, no manager, whether technical specialist or management generalist, is immune to inappropriate organizational behavior. Both generalist managers and technical-specialist managers can display self-serving tendencies at times. Some managers, however, frequently differ in how they pursue their objectives of service according to whether they see themselves as a generalist or as a technical specialist. The generalist who is on a self-serving track often tends toward empire building, working to acquire every function or responsibility that can in any way be connected under a common head. This manager is working toward elevation of self by acquiring far-reaching control throughout the organization, much as some nations formerly extended their authority by acquiring colonies throughout the world.

The self-serving technical specialist manager, however, is often limited by the inability to absorb functions that are not technically related to the profession of the manager. Rather than building an empire, this manager—much like the feudal baron who remained in his castle, but devoted most of his time and energies to making it the grandest and strongest castle in the country—strives to build an elegant structure that will surely dwarf its neighbors. Thus the "most important" specialty eventually has the most elegant quarters, the most generous budget, the most favorable staffing relative to the amount of work to be done, and the strongest voice in influencing organizational policy. The results convey the belief that one's own profession is somehow better than the other professions in the organization.

Example: A "Professional" Ego Problem

There is another ego problem to which the technical specialist manager may fall victim, one of perhaps significantly more impact than the effect just described. It is found in the tendency to place management in an inferior role relative to the profession, or to consider that the profession itself is somehow essential to management. The governing belief seems to be that one could not possibly become an accomplished manager without knowledge of this particular profession. A brief story may provide clarification.

A consortium of health care organizations agreed to cooperate in a joint undertaking to develop a comprehensive series of educational programs for health care managers. The members decided against following the more conventional practices for such activities, such as placing development solely in the hands of trainers and human resources people, and chose to involve a cross section of working health care managers. Due to sheer numbers it was not practical to structure this advisory body to include representatives from every profession or technical specialty in all of the consortium's member organizations, nor was much serious thought given to doing so. Although the resulting group included representatives from roughly one-half of the technical specialties found in a full-service hospital, some health care occupations were missing. This was seen as presenting no particular problem because the focus of the advisory group's activities was management. Every manager involved, whether technical specialist or pure generalist, was qualified in his or her primary field, but the group's interest would be specific to management, to those techniques and practices applicable in all settings to the business of getting things done through people.

However, the advisory group's composition was no sooner made public when the consortium received complaints from various specialist-managers who claimed that their occupations were "ignored," "obviously overlooked," or "shabbily treated by exclusion from the process." One individual suggested that the group's deliberations could produce little of value to health care managers in general because the group did not include a speech pathologist. Another, pointing out that one member of the group was a manager in diagnostic radiology, claimed the necessity to include a manager in therapeutic radiology to make the group's deliberations worthwhile. Still another expressed shock and dismay that the group did not include a social work manager and went so far as to claim that the field of social work had contributed more to the advancement of health care management than any other field.

The between-the-lines message received from the managers whose activities were not represented in the group came through loud and clear: My technical specialty is critically important in health care management. However, this is simply not true. As far as management is concerned, one's technical specialty is critically important only in the internal management of that technical specialty. No single technical specialty is critical in health care management in general. The knowledge and perspective of an individual profession are essential in making the professional judgments that are necessary, but only within the context of managing the technical work of that profession. To believe that one's base of technical expertise is somehow part of the foundation of management knowledge is an error of considerable magnitude. Such a belief is an ego-based reaction that causes one to elevate one's own specialty over others, and further to place it in a position of superiority over management. When this occurs, the individual is actually favoring the technical specialist hat and claiming that it is more important than the management hat.

Attempt to Subordinate Management

In truth, to be a well-rounded and effective health care manager one need not be a social worker, speech pathologist, laboratory technologist, registered nurse, respiratory therapist, or any other health care specialist. It is automatically conceded that in all but the most general of support activities the manager must be some kind of specialist as well as manager. (It certainly requires, for example, a physical therapist to oversee the work of other physical therapists.) However, no one particular specialty has a monopoly, or even a modest edge, regarding management expertise. The fundamental task of management—the business of getting things done through people—is reflected in practices such as proper delegation, clear and open two-way communication, budgeting and cost control, scheduling, handling employee problems, and applying disciplinary action. All true management practices are fully transportable across departmental lines, and to believe otherwise is to fall into the ego trap of the technical specialist.

Part of this ego effect is to place management in a subordinate position relative to the technical specialty. To conclude the foregoing tale about the consortium, a number of critics of the composition of the advisory group pointed out that management courses had been part of their education. This is indeed so; in their college education most health care professionals receive some classroom training, largely theoretical, in management and supervision. However, management courses constitute a small part of most health professionals' educational curricula. To assume that this relatively small amount of management theory is sufficient to prepare one to manage a department is indeed placing management in the back seat relative to the technical specialty.

As mentioned, the technical specialist who enters management is literally adopting a second career. If one wishes to think of management as a profession—and, to many, management is indeed a profession of considerable depth and breadth—then one must recognize the necessity to enter management with as much preparation as possible. Consider, for a moment, the reverse of the ego effect recently described. Imagine that a student of business administration managed to take three or four courses in sociology and social work (perhaps as electives) and after graduation claimed to be qualified as a social worker as well as a management generalist. It is highly unlikely that true technical specialists, especially social workers, would accept this individual's "instant expertise." Yet this same tendency to assume a capability for which one is unqualified is exhibited by, for example, the social worker who on the strength of two or three management courses lays claim to being qualified as a manager as well as a social worker.

Ego can provide massive barriers to one's effectiveness as a manager; massive because the person encountering such barriers rarely recognizes doing so. To a person with such an orientation, management is something that anyone can do. It suggests a belief that "I am smart enough to be a member of an important profession, so therefore I am more than smart enough to be a manager (perhaps not everyone can manage, but surely one as smart as I can manage)."

In summary, the ego barrier to managerial effectiveness consists of two important dimensions:

1. An inflated view of the importance of one's profession relative to the importance of management; and

2. The failure to recognize management, devoid of all implications of any other particular occupation, as a specialty in its own right.

The obstacles presented by ego are overcome with great difficulty. In many cases, perhaps the majority, they are never overcome. This is unfortunate because the most significant effects of the ego barrier are the tendency to place organizational interests second to department interests, and the proliferation and perpetuation of middle-management mediocrity.

TRANSFERENCE OF EXPERTISE

Occasionally the professional who is not a manager appears to be attempting to exercise an assumed competence in an area of endeavor without adequate preparation. This phenomenon—transference of expertise, discussed briefly with a somewhat different perspective in Chapter 5—occurs when a technical specialist, frequently a high-skill professional (quite often a physician), assumes a nonexistent capability in another activity, usually management. Though not articulated, the individual's behavior demonstrates the following rationale: "I am a doctor of medicine (or a dentist or a chemist, or whatever), and my field is obviously more difficult and more important than management. I know that my field is more important because it requires years of study to become qualified, whereas one can become a manager by simple organizational appointment and without special education. Therefore, not just anyone can practice in my field but anyone *can* indeed practice management. Management is a lesser function than my own, so if I can successfully practice my own specialty I must readily be able to manage—and manage better than most managers. I thus transfer my level of expertise to any field that is of lesser difficulty than my own specialty."

Physicians cannot be blamed for occasionally assuming a management expertise that may not be theirs. Medicine is a noble and difficult calling, and society has long deferred to its healers. When so many persons regard physicians as workers of wonders, it is understandable for some physicians to occasionally lose sight of their normal human limitations.

The anyone-can-do-it attitude toward management is by no means limited to physicians or other high-skill professionals. This attitude is reflected by many persons who may be educated to widely varying degrees and who work at jobs ranging from unskilled entry-level positions to highly skilled medical specialists, all of whom have but one factor in common: They have never been called on to manage, or at least have never yet run up against their limitations as managers. Regardless of background, the person entering management for the first time who is most likely to succeed is the person who accepts management as a distinctly separate career in its own right, with principles and techniques that must be studied, learned, and diligently practiced.

THE CHANGING STATE OF HEALTH CARE MANAGEMENT

Forces Affecting the Health care Manager

For more than three decades the American health care system has been under increasing pressure to change. For more than 30 years, health care costs have steadily risen at rates well beyond the rate of so-called normal inflation. External influences have been brought to bear on organizations that deliver health care, some intended to restrict the flow of financial resources into the system and some intended to limit the use of various services. The health care industry in general, and in certain major segments, specifically hospitals and other institutional providers, has reacted to a growing number of external influences with measures intended to improve their efficiency and ensure their financial viability.

The kinds of changes recently occurring in organized health care delivery are having significant effects on management at the departmental level. Because so many health care organization departments are overseen by professionals working as managers, the changes bearing on the system are directly affecting how the professional-as-manager must manage.

Work organizations have never been static entities; they have necessarily changed as their environments and missions and purposes have changed. For many years, however, organizational change did not necessarily simultaneously affect a great many functions at the departmental operating level. Recently, though, the changes affecting health care organizations have been felt in all functions, in all activities, and at all levels, and as a result department managers' roles are changing.

We have of course heard much about reengineering, and indeed this has been one of the major forces reshaping the department manager's role. Add to reengineering the increasing numbers of mergers and other affiliations occurring between and among provider organizations, and we are left with what are often dramatic changes to which the department manager must adjust.

Reengineering by Any Other Name

A probable majority of organizations call it "reengineering." A few might call it "repositioning." Some might still call it "downsizing," "rightsizing," or simply "reorganizing." Regardless of the label attached to the process, the intended result is the same: To reorder the processes by which the organization does its work to enable it to accomplish the right things with the least amount of resources. (And regardless of what it is called, to many employees, managers and nonmanagers alike, any name given to the reengineering process has the same meaning: some people are going to lose their jobs.)

True reengineering, beginning with a clear focus on desired output and working backward to determine how best to achieve that output, consumes large amounts of time and energy. It also frequently requires considerable amounts of money in the form of consultant costs and other expenses. But more often than not it is embarked upon when financial fortunes are waning and there is a perceived need to do something to stave off disaster.

There is often considerable apprehension in the manager's knowledge that "reengineering is coming." This is usually the fear that one's own position will be eliminated, a fear frequently borne out as reengineering proceeds. Faced with the reality of reengineering , as well as the ever-present possibility of job loss through merger or affiliation, today's health care department managers are hampered in three significant dimensions:

1. They are at risk, and this manifests itself as fear and uncertainty.

2. They cannot step back and objectively view that which intimately involves them because they are internal to the organization; they are part of the problem.

3. They are affected far more than they might ever be able to acknowledge because some long-held paradigms remain under concentrated—and largely successful—attack.

Organizational Flattening: Common Reengineering Fallout

An organization that grows fat—i.e., is complex, has too many levels, built-in entrenched bureaucracies—usually does so over an extended period of time. However, organizational flattening (the elimination and compression of layers of management) usually occurs abruptly. A structure that required years to develop may be taken down a level or two in a matter of weeks, or perhaps even days.

Organizational flattening is likely to remain a factor in health care for some time to come. With flattening comes genuine pain, dismay, disappointment, and perhaps a generous measure of fear. It also comes with lots of uncertainty about the future, and, as a result, strong feelings of insecurity where perhaps none previously existed.

The middle management level (the managers of the first-line managers) is often most vulnerable to organizational flattening. When organizational structures are compressed, more often than not middle managers either disappear or become first-line managers (or supervisors, as might be the term descriptive of first-line management).

Since organizational flattening involves the removal of one or more levels from the chain of command, it usually means that increased decision-making authority accrues to the first-line manager. Imagine a three-level hierarchy in which there is a middle manager between a first-line manager and a top manager. If the middle management position is eliminated, some of what the middle manager formerly did will no longer be done by anyone. (Often when a management level is eliminated, unnecessary or redundant tasks performed at that level become highly visible.) Some of what remains will be absorbed by the top manager, but most of the remaining essential work will fall to the first-line manager. When a hierarchy grows; that is, becomes fatter, decision-making authority and responsibility tend to be forced up the chain of command, with significant decisions made at increasingly higher levels. When a hierarchy shrinks, that is, becomes flattened, decision-making authority and responsibility tend to be forced downward. Therefore the flattened organization usually means that the first-line manager must take on greater responsibility and do so without middle management backup.

A flatter organization can also mean more responsibility for the first-line manager in the form of more employees to look after—that is, a greatly increased span of control—and thus more employee-related tasks to perform. This emphasizes the need to empower employees, to encourage them toward ownership of their jobs. To the first-line manager, flattening brings several "mores"—more people problems (because of more people), more specific responsibilities, more tasks to take on personally, and more coordination and communication needs. More of almost everything, except perhaps pay and benefits, although flattening reasonably accomplished may be accompanied by modest increases for the survivors who are expected to take on more work.

Sometimes two positions that have something in common are combined. This may occur in an organization that is experiencing shrinkage horizontally as well as vertically, and it may occur when two formerly separate organizations merge and their department management staffs are consolidated. Merger has in fact been a driver of many such consolidations; two institutions merge corporately into a single organization, like functions are combined, and a single manager is appointed over what is in effect a two-location department.

There are three common scenarios for consolidating the management of two groups into one:

1. One of the two present managers is chosen by higher management.

2. The two managers must compete with each other and outside candidates in an interview and selection process.

3. Both present managers are displaced and a new manager is recruited.

These choices should themselves emphasize how difficult shrinking an organization or merging organizations can be for middle and lower management. In even the kindest of these scenarios, one of the present managers loses out; in the others, one or both can lose out. In fact it is not unusual for the process to focus on outside candidates only, as someone who does not come from one of the existing groups will not be wedded to a former way of doing things.

Change as a Way of Life

Rapid technological change in medicine continues, making a strong technical orientation all the more important for the individual manager. Now more than ever the manager will have to strive to stay current technologically as well as managerially. The two hats will each remain equally important, and because of changes on both sides of the job—structural, organizational, and functional changes affecting the management role, as well as technological changes affecting the specialist role—the manager will experience intensifying pressure on both sides.

A Look Ahead

Over the coming decade or so, the professional-as-manager working in health care delivery is likely to experience

- continued difficulty in filling essential jobs;
- increased staffing and scheduling difficulties that will be addressed in part by greater reliance on alternative scheduling practices (part-timers, flextime, job sharing, and so forth); and
- increased sensitivity to employee rights, as legislation governing the employment relationship continues to expand.

Overall, what the health care manager of the near future can expect is an increasing amount of challenge, and thus significant opportunity for learning and growth and for a greatly increased sense of accomplishment.

QUESTIONS AND ACTIVITIES

1. Fully explain why the professional employee is likely to experience more difficulty than the nonprofessional in balancing the two sides of the management role.

2. Thoroughly describe a set of circumstances under which it would seem advantageous to recruit a new manager from outside rather than promoting an internal candidate.

3. Using examples as appropriate, explain what is meant by describing management as a "soft" science.

4. Fully explain why management is frequently not regarded as a profession in its own right.

5. Management as a profession is different from all other professions in one critical dimension. Describe this dimension.

6. Thoroughly describe a set of circumstances under which it would seem advantageous to promote an internal candidate rather than recruiting a new manager from outside the organization.

7. A significant number of people seem to harbor the attitude that management is something that "anyone can do." Explain why this attitude can develop, highlighting the characteristics of management that might support this belief.

QUESTIONS AND ACTIVITIES *(continued)*

8. In some instances of merging two organizations, the decision has been made to remove both existing managers or administrators and recruit a new leader from outside of both organizations. Describe both the advantages and disadvantages of this practice.

9. Following the merger of two institutions located several miles apart, the professional functions at both were merged under common heads. In other words, for each professional function one manager was removed and one was given the combined responsibility. Describe the more obvious ways in which the management role has changed for the surviving manager.

10. Frequently management's greatest critics, including those who believe that management is something "anyone can do," are those who have never managed. Explain why this is so.

11. Considering the professional-as-manager, provide two to three examples of situations in which the professional or technical side of the role must be allowed to temporarily dominate.

12. Fully explain why a professional working as a manager might begin in management by strongly favoring the "technical hat," but gradually drift toward chronically favoring the "management hat."

13. Imagine an organization that implemented an extensive total quality management (TQM) undertaking but has most recently decided upon a reengineering effort that is likely to result in staff reductions. Identify and explain the critical contradiction that is bound to arise when reduction-in-force follows TQM.

14. Describe one instance in which "transference of expertise" may be at least partially justified or may be legitimate to some extent.

15. The statement of *The Peter Principle* is: *In a hierarchy every employee tends to rise to his level of incompetence* (*The Peter Principle*, Laurence J. Peter and Raymond Hull, William Morrow and Company, Inc., 1969). Explain how this effect might seem descriptive of some technical professionals who accept promotion to management positions.

CHAPTER 11

Unionization and the Professional

The trade unionist has the same limitation imposed upon him as the capitalist. He cannot advance his interests at the expense of society.
—J. Ramsay MacDonald

This Chapter Will:

► Review the present state of union organizing within the health care industry, especially as concerns professional employees;

► Highlight the fundamental management errors that most often cause employees to turn to labor unions;

► Outline the health care organization's primary areas of vulnerability to union organizing;

► Explore the key role ideally fulfilled by the first-line manager whose employees are undergoing union organizing;

► Comment briefly on decertification, the process by which a unionized group of employees can shed union representation.

THE ORGANIZING EMPHASIS IN HEALTH CARE

A Growing Problem for Health Care Management

When considering union organizing activity nationwide across all industry lines, it is not difficult to conclude that the rate at which unions are winning representation elections is steadily decreasing. On average, a target employer's chance of remaining union-free after a representation election is probably greater than it has been in more than 30 years. Coupled with this decreasing rate of union victories is a change in how the unions are faring in decertification elections, those relatively few elections held specifically to decide the issue of removing union representation. The proportion of union victories in decertification elections is declining; that is, a growing number of employee groups are voting in favor of removing the unions they had earlier voted into power.

In addition, unionized workers are declining as a percentage of the country's workforce. Total union membership in all American industries combined has shown a steady decline from approximately 20 percent of the workforce in 1983 to 13.5 percent of the workforce in 2001, the lowest level of union membership since the passage of the National Labor Relations Act in 1935. When workers belonging to public employee unions are excluded, unions represent less than 10 percent of workers in the private sector.[1]

Much of the unions' membership losses are attributable to the decline in numbers of jobs available in manufacturing, the original and long-time stronghold of organized labor. Since 1979, jobs in the service sector of the economy have grown by more than 50 percent, to where they now represent more than 80 percent of American jobs, while manufacturing jobs declined more than 10 percent.[2] During 2000 it was stated that organized labor had to add 250,000 to 500,000 members every year to keep up with the losses generated by job attrition in manufacturing.[3]

Does this mean that unions are simply going away, and that management should regard them as less of a threat than they once were? Nothing could be further from the truth. If anything, unions, especially in the health care industry, are more of a threat than ever.

Many people think of unions almost exclusively in terms of heavy manufacturing industry, or in terms of shipping or transportation activities such as trucking or loading and unloading cargo ships. It is certainly true that widespread unionization was long the pattern throughout manufacturing and certain other heavily labor intensive activities. However, manufacturing and other traditional union stronghold industries such as mining have been steadily losing workers for three to four decades. Many of these losses are permanent for all practical purposes as the American economy continues to shift away from heavy manufacturing toward areas of high technology and human services. This loss of workers to industry means a loss of members to unions.

In the face of declining membership unions are struggling to maintain their relevance, and they are actively looking for potential members in areas that have traditionally been nonunion, or that have been only partly organized. One can see organizing efforts—and union victories—in industries thought of as essentially nonunion, such as banking, insurance, retailing, and health care. Unions are concentrating heavily on health care and on high-tech areas, and it is no stretch of the imagination to recognize that many health care professionals fall under both headings—health care and high-tech.

Whether viewed by manufacturing or transportation unions attempting to branch out, or by established white-collar or professional unions attempting to do the same, health care appears as an inviting organizing target. Health care employees in general, and hospital employees in particular are highly desired by unions. Health care was for a considerable time viewed as an expanding industry and an expanding labor market, making it an attractive organizing target. Some elements of health care, specifically hospitals, appear to be shrinking as employers rather than expanding, but health care overall continues to expand as the population grows and much health care delivery moves into settings other than the acute-care hospital. When the unions view health care they see large numbers of employees whose wages are generally increasing, and who could become a significant source of dues. They also see numerous provider organizations bending under financial pressures and giving way to changes in health care delivery, with some organizations, again primarily hospitals, going out of business. Other organizations enter into mergers and other affiliations, resulting in large numbers of health care employees who feel insecure in their employment.

There appears to be no end in sight for what many would describe as the turmoil in health care. In the face of mounting layoffs arising from mergers and acquisitions, and other affiliations and cutbacks made in response to growing financial pressure, many health care workers are taking a second look at unions and the unions are encouraging them to do so. Health care management's often desperate efforts to achieve and maintain solvency have affected relations with employees. Employees are growing steadily more unhappy and insecure, and insecurity pushes employees toward unions.

Within health care, union activity has increased steadily since the 1975 amendments to the National Labor Relations Act extended the coverage of that act to employees of nonprofit hospitals. Unions that had their beginnings in nonhealth activities have expanded into health care, and other unions still associated with vastly different industries are making inroads into health care as well. Certain organizations that began as professional associations have become collective bargaining organizations representing members of specific occupational groups. Examples of unions active in health care are as follows:

- The Service Employees International Union (SEIU), which represents perhaps 300,000 or more health care employees;
- The National Union of Hospital and Health Care Employees, District 1199 (commonly known as "1199"), a division of the Retail, Wholesale, and Department Store Union, which represents perhaps 150,000 health care workers;
- The American Federation of Teachers, through a division known as the Federation of Nurses and Health Professionals;
- The various state affiliates of the American Nurses' Association (ANA), formerly a straightforward professional association; and
- Various locals of the Teamsters, the Communications Workers of American (CWA), and other unions formerly associated exclusively with nonhealth industries.

None of the foregoing—and none of the various other unions courting health care workers—are to be taken lightly. For example, even in the face of declining union victories overall, the state affiliates of the American Nurses' Association continues to win the majority of the representation elections in which it is involved.

Health care offers large numbers of potential members for unions. Also, health care is easily the most heavily regulated industry in the country, with no end to the increasing regulatory pressure in sight. With regulation come additional constraints and demands, with constraints and demands comes increasing frustration, and with frustration comes employee dissatisfaction. Much of this regulation is of course financial in nature. Although health care wages have increased dramatically over their pathetic levels of the past—it was only as recent as 1967 that hospital workers were afforded the minimum wage coverage provided by the Fair Labor Standards Act—some health care workers are not yet on pay scales fully equivalent to their nonhealth counterparts. In these times of health care cost control, a health institution's dollars go just so far, and many health care workers who spend each day working with half-million dollar machines in multimillion dollar structures at the beck and call of highly paid physicians hear themselves told that there is insufficient money left for raises this year.

In short, much of health care is seen as ripe for union organizing—and the unions, many of which always welcome new members and more than a few of which need new members to offset massive losses, are more than willing to fill the void. It may indeed be clear that unions are on the decline as a percentage of the total work force. However, it should be equally clear that union organizing in health care is on the increase and is likely to intensify for some time to come.

The Professional Employee

The definition of *professional* in the National Labor Relations Act (NLRA) is nearly the same as that in the Fair Labor Standards Act (FLSA). That is, according to the NLRA a *professional* is one whose work

- is predominantly intellectual (as opposed to routine);
- involves independent judgment;
- is not susceptible to standardization; and
- requires knowledge acquired through prolonged study in an institution of higher learning or in a hospital.

Many health care professionals are clearly of the opinion that union membership runs counter to professionalism, and that it somehow makes one less of a professional to belong to a union. This belief constitutes a strong force in an industry that has become known as a stronghold of professionalism. On the other hand, many health care professionals feel that unions support professional unity and are necessary to offset what they see as management's shortcomings. Recent years have seen many health care professionals turning to unions for representation because

- they have come to believe that organization is the only way they have to be clearly heard and to influence change affecting their roles in health care; and

- they are reacting to difficult economic times and to health care cost containment, and feel that the spiraling increase in health care costs is being addressed at least in part at their expense by keeping their numbers lean and their salaries in check.

Recent years' activity in health care has revealed that workers are inclined to be bolder in labor activities when their skills are in short supply. In many parts of the country this has certainly been the case with nurses. Given the declining enrollments in nursing schools and the dropout rate for the profession, the available supply of nurses in many areas has not kept pace with expanding demand. Those working nurses who are needed, and know that they are needed, can hardly be blamed for attempting to improve the conditions of their employment. Nurses, however, are far from being the only group of interest to labor organizers.

For many years the kinds of bargaining units—the groupings of workers considered for representation purposes—were defined by precedent. It was common, for example, for all of the nonexempt employees in a hospital to be represented by a single union, but it was just as common for two or three or even four unions to represent different groups of workers within the same institution. One of the intents of the United States Congress in framing the 1975 amendments to the NLRA was to avoid fragmentation of bargaining units; that is, to keep the number of different unions that could represent workers in the same organization to a practical minimum. However, regardless of the congressional intent in the late 1980s the National Labor Relations Board (NLRB) acted in essentially the opposite direction. Rules issued by the NLRB, and eventually upheld by the United States Supreme Court, officially designated eight (8) bargaining units as appropriate in acute-care hospitals. Still applicable in the present decade, these are

- Registered nurses
- Physicians
- All other professionals
- Technical employees
- Skilled maintenance employees
- Business office clerical employees
- Security officers
- All other nonprofessional employees (service workers, etc.)

When a union representation election is in the offing, management and the union jointly decide on unit boundaries unless the courts or some federal agency intervene. Ordinarily the union states the unit it wants, and the employer either negotiates the unit boundaries with the union or appeals to the NLRB or to the courts.

The NLRA prevents the Board from placing professionals and nonprofessionals in the same unit unless the majority of the professionals vote in favor of such inclusion. Some specialists—a relative few—can request professional exemption from a unit that includes both professional and nonprofessional employees. If not among the select few eligible for exemption, some professional workers may be counted as in a given bargaining unit whether or not they wish to be included. (The exceptions are the few states that have right-to-work laws, which make the closed shop—compulsary union membership as a condition of employment—illegal.)

These references to professionals pertain, according to the NLRB, to "nurses, physicians, and other professionals." The Board's list of professionals, certainly not to be considered all-inclusive, is:

- Audiologists
- Cardiopulmonary technologists
- Chemists
- Dieticians
- Educational programmers
- Medical artists
- Medical technologists
- Mental health clinicians
- Pulmonary functions technologists

- Physical and occupational therapists
- Radiologic paramedics
- Recreation therapists
- Speech therapists
- Teachers

Prohibitions against including certain professionals in certain units notwithstanding, the health care organizations undergoing union organizing can usually expect frequent disputes over unit boundaries. For example, the NLRB position has long been that a separate unit of registered nurses—that is, separate from other professionals—is always proper. However, in spite of NLRB guidelines some courts have held that a separate registered nurse unit ignores the original congressional mandate to avoid proliferation of bargaining units. On this basis some courts have ordered other professionals included with nurses, especially in smaller organizations in which there may be but a relative handful of "other professionals." This question of unit boundaries will likely continue to be an issue for some time to come, with some specific instances resolved only by court decision.

Nurses make up the largest group of health care professionals, and to date they continue to be the most militant as far as organizing is concerned. If the other-professionals unit boundary issue eventually goes solidly in the direction of fewer bargaining units, nearly all of the professionals in any given health care organization could find themselves swept along with the nurses. Because of sheer numbers, the nurses would dominate the choice of representation for all professionals in the organization.

As most other workers who organize, the professional employee is seeking economic security and job satisfaction. But also as others who organize, the professional often finds that a measure of economic security can be attained—but that job satisfaction remains elusive, not attainable by virtue of a legal contract.

Economics forever remain important to workers—all workers, at all levels—who may be inclined to organize. For professional employees, however, other matters remain fully as important as economics—matters of career, professionalism, and even lifestyle.

The Unique Position of the Professional Nurse

In recent years there has been increasing unrest among nurses, and considerably more focus on organizing for collective bargaining, as nurses attempt to use collective action to advance their aims and enhance their status. As mentioned, there is increasing pressure to include nurses in bargaining units with all other professionals. This is not yet a common practice, but should it become common then by their sheer numbers nurses would be in a position to move virtually all of an institution's professionals into a union whether or not the other professionals want to.

Although hospital nurses in general appear to be strongly divided on the subject of labor unions as the best means to attain and retain professional status, they are by and large united in their dedication to professionalism and patient care. Any force that appears to bear the potential to weaken professionalism is regarded with caution, and any perceived threats to professionalism are opposed regardless of where they come from (union, administration, government, or elsewhere). Activity during the closing decades of the twentieth century essentially confirmed the rapid spread of collective bargaining among those nurses who believe that there is no other way to achieve their goals regarding status, professionalism, and patient care. Still, on the question of compatibility of unionization with professionalism, registered nurses remain divided. Some go so far as to claim that unions are the best thing to happen to nursing in the modern era, a feeling among nurses that seems to have been growing steadily since health care, and especially hospitals, first began to feel the pinch of cost control in the late 1960s.

Even though a significant percent of professional nurses favor collective bargaining, many express serious reservations about strikes and other forms of work stoppage. Also, many are of the opinion that a union for nurses can be professional only if it is organized by nursing personnel, and only if nurses are represented for collective bargaining purposes by nurses only. Thus even among nurses who readily accept unionization as a way to achieve their goals, many continue to prefer representation by professional nursing associations. Nevertheless, many pro-union nurses have collectively expressed the opinion that their nursing management and the leaders of the American Nurses' Association and its affiliated state organizations are not adequately representing nurses.

To nurses who express an anti-union posture, unions do not appear to be the way to enhance their status and professionalism. These people generally identify collective bargaining with factory workers and tradespeople, and thus they tend to regard unions as philosophically contrary to the concept of a profession. The strongest support for unions of professional nurses tends to come from younger nurses, while a majority of older nurses, those in mid-career or beyond, seem to believe there is basic incompatibility between unionism and professionalism.

It should be clear, however, that nurses today are actively seeking genuine recognition of their professionalism as nurses and their status as key members of the health care delivery team. It follows that the organizing bodies with the best chances of capturing the membership, support, and loyalty of a portion of the nurses not yet organized are those groups that place the recognition or professionalism clearly over and above attention to programs and promises.

Managers and Unions

In view of what is happening with some nurses and even with some physicians and other health care professionals, the longstanding belief that one's status as a so-called professional indicates a predisposition to spurn membership in collective bargaining units is swiftly becoming a thing of the past. It can no longer be assumed (if indeed it were ever reasonable to assume so) that because one is a professional, one is automatically opposed to unionization. However, top management groups of many health care organizations continue to operate on the implicit assumption that a person's status as a member of management carries with it automatic opposition to unions. Indeed, in numerous counter-organizing campaigns top management groups have paid dearly for operating under the assumption that all supervisors and middle managers are philosophically opposed to collective arrangements and thus guaranteed to be on the side of management.

In many work organizations and particularly in large, far-reaching bureaucratic structures, lower and middle management attitudes toward labor organization extend beyond mere acceptance and passive support of collective bargaining units for their employees. A surprisingly high proportion of such management employees can be found to harbor thoughts of active participation in collective bargaining. Past surveys of managers have suggested that a significant percent of first-line and middle managers would join a manager's union if it were available, or they would consider doing so if they first approved of the union's philosophy and organizational structure.

All managers are not necessarily on the same side as top management regarding unionization. Much of what can be said about middle management is the same as what many are saying today about professional employees. Specifically, that middle management frustration and discontent are increasing, particularly because of prevailing working conditions, decreasing economic and job security, and a declining sense of personal realization and achievement in their jobs.

VULNERABILITY TO UNION ORGANIZING

No employer is invulnerable to union organizing. For management to believe so is a form of smugness that represents a considerable measure of vulnerability. Even union officials will concede that it takes an organization treating its employees poorly or thoughtlessly to form a union. In other words, no union can readily organize a contented workforce.

Vulnerability is relative to a number of factors. However, experience has shown that organizing drives—most originating inside the organization as employees reach out for representation—usually stem from employee dissatisfaction with some or all of the following:

Quality of Direct Supervision

Quality of supervision is a key factor for all employees whether professional or nonprofessional. The organization may be vulnerable if

- insufficient attention is given to placing managers out of consideration for communications skills, leadership, and problem-solving abilities and the like (as opposed to making placement decisions based on technical skills alone);
- there is little or no emphasis placed on management development;
- top management fails to act on apparent supervisory weaknesses (discrimination, harassment, favoritism, neglect, and so on); and
- no effort is made to stimulate and promote upward communication, and no readily accessible channels are open to employees.

Organizational Stability and Job Security

The organization may be vulnerable if

- there are frequent, surprise shifts in workload and work distribution;
- there is a history of instability, leading the employees to anticipate periodic layoffs;
- there is no rational, consistent approach to layoff, recall, and bumping;
- surprise changes occur in job structure and assignments;
- new methods and new equipment are introduced without advance notice; and
- minimal information is provided about opportunities for advancement or training and development.

Compensation and Benefits

The organization may be vulnerable if

- pay rates are not comparable with other health care organizations and other relevant competitors;
- there is no reflection of individual performance in the granting of raises;
- there are internal inequities in pay;
- employees do not understand how their pay is determined;
- there is no job evaluation program or other systematic approach to grading jobs and thus for setting rates of pay;
- employees are dissatisfied with their benefit plans as compared with the plans of competitors and other local employers;
- arbitrary changes in benefits occur by surprise; and
- employees lack knowledge of the details of their benefit programs.

Input to Organizational Processes

For this area of concern of particular importance to professional employees, the organization may be vulnerable if

- employees feel they have no input into the form and structure of their jobs and/or no voice in how their work is done;
- employees feel that they have no say regarding decisions that affect them; and
- employees receive no management response to their suggestions, problems, and questions.

Problem Resolution Process

The organization may be vulnerable if

- discipline is not applied fairly, uniformly, and consistently;
- disciplinary actions are taken without extending employees a reasonable opportunity to correct their behavior;
- there is no formal, consistent, multistep problem or grievance resolution procedure; and
- recent disciplinary actions are generally perceived as inconsistent, arbitrary, or unfair.

Working Conditions and Facilities

The organization may be vulnerable if

- hazardous or unpleasant tasks or physical areas are not addressed and controlled;
- there is no formal safety program and no apparent attention given to employee safety; and
- there is widespread dissatisfaction with physical facilities and employee services (cafeteria service, food quality, parking, temperature control, workplace décor, and so on).

Selection and Placement

The organization may be vulnerable if

- there is no written and observed policy regarding equal employment opportunity (EEO) and other fair employment practices;
- any job categories appear to be segregated according to race, gender, creed, and so forth; and
- employment application forms do not meet all regulatory requirements, and personnel representatives and supervisors are not fully trained in the proper preemployment questions that can or cannot legally be asked.

Employee Morale

The organization may be vulnerable if

- there is general failure to maintain constant awareness of possible problems in employee attitude; and
- there is general failure to maintain an active interest in employee morale, even at times when there are no apparent problems.

The extent of how vulnerable an organization may be to union organizing will depend to a considerable degree on how many of the foregoing represent actual points of dissatisfaction. How many does it take? On how many issues, practices, or policies must an organization be vulnerable before the union organizers have the edge? No one can say; it depends entirely on what factors are of most importance to any particular employee group, and how strongly the employees feel about any particular issue or problem. It should go without saying, however, that the more positive the organization comes across overall, the less vulnerable it will be to union organizing.

THE ORGANIZING APPROACH

What do the first stages of a union organizing campaign look like? One might be inclined to answer this question by citing one of the first visible signs: leafleting, or the distribution of union literature to employees at walkways, driveways, and parking lot entrances. Although serious leafleting is an undeniable indication of union activity, it is ordinarily not the first step in a union organizing campaign. Chances are that the union has been studying the organization for weeks, or even months, to judge its organizing potential before the first literature appears out in the open. (Specifically targeted groups of employees may have been receiving printed matter from the union for quite some time before any literature appears publicly.)

When organizing activity actually begins, management may know nothing about it. In fact, during the earliest stages the union may take considerable precautions to prevent management from learning about its interest. The union may send organizers into the facility simply to loiter and listen, in an effort to pick up what they can from conversations in the cafeteria, snack bar, parking areas, employee lounge areas, and other places where employees congregate informally. Outsiders can move around freely in many facilities, and such infiltration is especially easy in an institution that does not enforce the use of employee identification badges or passes for visitors and vendors. The organizers simply merge with the crowd and listen, picking up gripes, locating supervisory weaknesses and departments with obvious morale problems, and identifying informal leaders among the employees. They try to learn as much as possible about the organization before revealing themselves.

The still unannounced organizers also attempt to pinpoint employees who have the potential to serve as internal organizers, looking especially for those employees who are popular, knowledgeable, reasonably articulate, and in some way unhappy with the organization.

Should their silent survey raise serious doubts that the institution could possibly be unionized, the organizers might simply withdraw without ever making their presence known. However, if they believe that the union stands a reasonable chance of succeeding, they are likely to identify themselves to a few selected employees and begin preparations to carry their message to others. Leafleting may well begin at this stage.

The major exception to the usual significance of leafleting occurs in a practice sometimes referred to as a *pass-through*. In a pass-through, the union devotes a day or two to distributing literature at perhaps several institutions in the same geographic area. There are generally cold visits—no preinvestigation has taken place. The union simply passes through the area and drops as much literature as possible with the employees of as many institutions as they can readily reach and follows up only if they receive expressions of interest from employees (the pass-through literature usually includes a reply card that can be returned for more information).

When the organizers are out in the open and their purpose is generally known, they step up their activities in meeting with employees and contacting them in other ways. Somewhere along the way, possibly through sympathetic employees, they attempt to obtain a list of names and addresses of all the facility's nonmanagerial employees. The union most certainly contacts many individual employees by telephone and seeks to visit the homes of others.

In talking with employees, the union attempts to uncover issues to use as rallying points for employee sympathy and support. The organizers attempt to identify martyrs and victims of "the system" and effectively play on emotions in spotlighting incidents of alleged unfair treatment and discrimination.

The union organizers go to great lengths to impress employees of their right to be treated as individuals. This may seem elementary because most of us express strong belief in the rights of the individual. If, however, in the face of seemingly indifferent management the union organizer is the first person to tell them this, then the ground for union credibility may exist. The organizers make every effort to develop a communicating relationship with the employees. This should sound familiar because the development of such a relationship is an essential part of the role of the manager.

Most issues and incidents brought to light by the union are specially selected to make management look bad. Lacking sufficient factual material, organizers frequently stage incidents intended to make the union look good and management look foolish. The manager's awareness of this particular organizing tactic is critical; it is all too easy to make an inappropriate statement or incorrect decision when confronted with a trumped-up grievance or problem at an inconvenient time and under awkward circumstances (which usually includes the presence of some employee witnesses). Such matters would be rightly dealt with by administration, labor relations, or whoever else may be coordinating the organization's counter-organizing activities. However, there is often the need for the manager to react on the spot, without making promises or commitments and without seeming to be refusing to listen to an employee. Afterward the incident can be promptly reported to the proper persons.

THE FIRST-LINE MANAGER'S KEY ROLE

We have talked about the importance of the manager–employee relationship. The individual manager is almost always the member of management whom the employees in the department know best. This person may indeed be the only member of the mysterious entity called management who most of the department's employees know on a first-name basis, or even know on speaking terms. Thus as employees see this manager, so too are they likely to see all of management and the organization itself. If they see management as unconcerned, uncaring, distant, or indifferent, that is likely how they will see the organization as a whole.

It follows then that the manager is in a key position when dealing with the threat of unionization. The individual manager is the link that ties a number of employees to higher management and thus to the organization. The manager's long-term behavior has a great deal to do with whether the department is a fertile ground for union organizing activity, and the manager's conduct and actions during a union organizing campaign exert a significant influence on the employees' reaction to the organizing drive.

By law, employees have the right to organize and the institution has the right to work within legal boundaries to remain union-free. The contest, however, is somewhat one-sided in that the conduct of the employer—and of the employer's representatives—is subject to far more scrutiny than the conduct of the union.

The manager's introduction to preventive labor relations should begin with thorough orientation of the pitfalls of behavior to be avoided. Although the rules are many, they fall into a simply described mode of behavior; what the manager cannot do during a union organizing campaign is captured in the TIPS rule (or SPIT, or PITS—whichever is most easily remembered). During union organizing the manager may not

- *threaten* employees, perhaps with possible loss of employment or other consequences;
- *interrogate* employees about their union activities or sympathies;
- *promise* employees favored treatment or other rewards for opposing the union; and
- *spy* on employees to determine their involvement in union activities.

A list of more complete, specific prohibitions appears in Exhibit 11–1. Despite the length of this list of examples, however, one can readily see that each specific prohibition relates to one of the four TIPS—threaten, interrogate, promise, or spy.

When considered within the context of Exhibit 11–1, the prohibitions may seem somewhat overwhelming. However, for very nearly every *cannot* there is a *can*—and then some. (See Exhibit 11–2.) All of the items on this list avoid violating the TIPS prohibition. Note one extremely important consideration: Although it is true that the manager cannot ask about union interest and activity, the manager can listen to anything that the employees volunteer. The

Exhibit 11–1   Examples of What the Manager *Cannot* Do During Union Organizing

1. Grant pay increases or make promises of rewards or special concessions if employees reject the union.

2. Threaten, discipline, or intimidate employees who become involved in union activity, or who demonstrate a willingness to accept the union.

3. Questions employees about organizing activities, union matters, or their involvement with the union. Employees may volunteer such information and the manager may listen, but the manager must not ask.

4. Visit the homes of employees to encourage them to oppose the union. (The union may visit employees' homes, but management may not.)

5. Attend union meetings or have favored employees do so to report back, or otherwise engage in undercover activities, to determine who is involved in union activities.

6. Prevent employees who are functioning as internal organizers from soliciting employee interest in the union during nonworking time (e.g., lunch and official breaks).

7. Threaten that adoption of the union will force the organization to lay off employees, reduce benefits, close, relocate, and so on.

8. Discriminate against employees who support the union in terms of promotions, demotions, layoffs, work assignments, disciplinary actions, and the like.

9. Furnish financial support to employees who agree to oppose the union, or be involved in encouraging petitions or other actions intended to convince employees to reject the union.

10. Ask prospective employees about past union affiliations. (This is is always prohibited during the employment process, whether or not a union is actively organizing.)

11. Make totally exclusive statements concerning the organization's position on unions; for example, "this institution will never deal with a union." This can be generalized as: Never say *never* in any statements or predictions about present or future dealings with a union.

12. Deviate from established policies or alter accepted practices for the purpose of disciplining or eliminating an employee who favors the union.

13. Use outside parties to threaten or coerce or otherwise try to influence employees to oppose the union.

14. Ask employees whether they have signed union authorization cards, or ask them how they intend to vote concerning the union.

implications of this are far-reaching, for it is the manager who has cultivated interpersonal skills and has become a sympathetic, nonthreatening listener who is readily made aware of what is going on in the department.

When asked, how should the manager go about explaining why he or she believes a union is neither needed nor desired? One can always fall back on a list such as that of Exhibit 11–2—the *can-do* list—and perhaps reinforce some

Exhibit 11–2 Examples of What the Manager *Can Do* During Union Organizing

1. Bar external organizers—that is, people who are not employed by the institution—from the institution's premises.

2. Give employees management's opinions about unions, including their policies and leaders, even in unfavorable terms.

3. Provide employees with factual information about the union and its officials, even if such information is unfavorable.

4. Actively campaign against a union that is attempting to represent employees, and respond to union criticism of the organization's policies and practices.

5. Remind employees of their legal right to participate or not participate in union activities as they so choose, and respond to their questions about the union's apparent expectations of them.

6. Inform employees of the disadvantages of union membership, such as strikes, dues, fines and assessment, and possible domination by a national or international union.

7. Inform employees that signing a union authorization card is neither a vote for the union nor a commitment to vote for the union.

8. Remind employees of the benefits they receive without a union, and advise them of how what they receive compares with what employees at other institutions are receiving.

9. Let employees know that management would prefer to deal with them directly rather than attempting to communicate through a third party.

10. Insist that all organizing activity be conducted outside of working time and away from exposure to the institution's patients.

11. Correct any false or misleading statements made by union organizers.

12. Declare management's opposition to compulsory union membership contracts (i.e., its opposition to contracts that force all employees to join the union whether or not it is their wish to do so).

13. Advise employees that despite union promises, the union cannot obtain more for them than the institution is able to give.

14. Advise employees that the organization may legally replace any employee who engages in a strike for economic reasons (i.e., strikes for increased pay or benefits).

of these by providing the employees with the constitution and bylaws of the particular organizing union. (This often serves to reveal the undemocratic nature of many of the union's processes.) However, for a simple, compelling rationale for avoiding membership in a collective bargaining organization, the manager might simply refer to the employees' basic communicating relationship with and without a union.

Refer to Figure 11–1. The simpler diagram—without union—is the basic communicating relationship in the manager–employee relationship. Communication flows, or at least it should flow, directly from one person to another. The supervisor or manager who has established the proper relationship with each employee works to keep the channel open and information flowing. When effort is put into making this one-to-one relationship work, the benefits of that effort are direct and visible and have full impact.

Figure 11–1 The Essential Communicating Relationship

Without Union

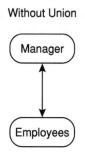

With Union

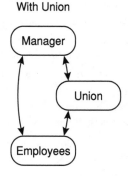

Consider the full implications of the second diagram—"with union"—for the manager–employee relationship. The presence of the union has caused a third party to be interjected into the manager–employee relationship, and in many ways this is no longer a clean communicating relationship. It is true that information flows between manager and employee, but only *some* information. Certain other items of information must now flow through the third party, and it is fundamental to organizational communication that the more levels or layers through which information must pass, the greater the chances of distortion and delay.

Also—and this is a critical consideration—the third-party in this three-way relationship is not a neutral party whose role is to ensure effective communication. Rather, this third party has selfish interests of its own to attend to. In theory the union exists to represent the employees. However, to be successful at being allowed to do so, the union must make the employees feel that there is reason for the union to represent them. No reason equals no need, no need often equals no union. An effective communicating relationship is based largely on mutual trust. A union, to justify its continued presence—and to justify the costs of membership and the privileges of the union's leadership—must foster sufficient distrust and discontent to prove continually that it is "needed" to represent the employees.

It is to the manager's advantage—at all times, but especially during a union organizing campaign—to know the employees as individuals and know them well. Although people cannot be stereotyped and there are few reliable generalizations concerning employees' receptiveness to a union, it is nevertheless possible to make some reasonable judgments as to how certain employees might react under organizing pressure. Often the employee who is sympathetic to the union cause may

- feel unfairly treated by the organization and believe that reasonable work opportunities have been denied;
- feel that the organization has been unsympathetic regarding personal problems and pressures;
- express a lack of confidence in management and be unwilling to talk openly with members of management;
- feel unequally treated in terms of pay and other economic benefits;
- take no apparent pride in affiliation with the institution;
- exhibit career path problems, having either changed jobs frequently or having reached the top in pay and classification while still having a significant number of working years remaining;

- be a source of complaints or grievances more often than most other employees; and

- exhibit a poor overall attitude.

It is extremely important for the manager to know the employees' attitudes toward the institution; the manager must develop a keen sense for how well he or she is communicating. Ultimately a labor union has little to offer if employees already feel that the organization is responding to their needs.

It is also important to appreciate that the best time to learn how to deal with a union organizing drive is before one occurs, and that as far as the institution's management is concerned, the key player is the first-line manager—that member of management who supervises the people who do the hands-on work.

THE BARGAINING ELECTION

The union, using both outside and inside organizers, goes about the business of securing sufficient employee interest to allow them to petition the NLRB for a representation election. Generally the indications of such support take the form of simple cards that employees sign to indicate interest in having an election. Employees should be aware that signing a card is not an automatic yes vote for union representation, but simply an expression of interest in having an election. Managers should make certain that their employees are aware of the true meaning of a signature card: Often when organizing is underway, organizers will pressure employees for their signatures and sometimes deliberately leave individuals with the impression that signing a card obligates them to vote in favor of the union. Some employees will sign cards simply to stop the organizers from pestering and pressuring them, so they need to know that signing a card—which some may regret having done—does not commit them to a "yes"vote.

When a sufficient number of signatures of employees in the unit that the union is seeking to represent are gathered (usually half or more—but at least 30 percent, per NLRB requirements), the union petitions the NLRB. After what is usually a cursory investigation, the board sanctions an election and a date for voting is set.

Election is by secret ballot, and all employees who work in the unit that the union is seeking to represent are eligible to vote. If the union receives a simple majority of the vote, it is then certified by the NLRB as the legal bargaining agent for all persons who work in the unit. Although compulsory union membership is not a legal requirement, this often means that all persons working in the unit must eventually join the union because this particular right of the union is usually bargained for in the initial contract. (The exceptions are the few right-to-work states where closed-shop contracts are forbidden.) If the union fails to achieve a simple majority and various possible legal challenges do not upset the results of the election, the union withdraws, at least for a while if the votes were close, or perhaps for a longer period if the results were clearly one-sided against the union.

It should be kept in mind, however, that some elections are little more than formalities—many elections are lost by management long before the organizers ever appear on the scene. If the trend in relations between employees and management is clearly in the direction of a union, this can be difficult to reverse, especially during the relatively limited time consumed by an organizing campaign. Reversal, however, may be accomplished through hard work and plenty of open and honest communication.

Even if a single unit of employees is lost to a union (e.g., a union representing registered nurses only, or security officers only), new steps aimed at creating positive communicating relationships can still pay off. A new atmosphere can make contract negotiations easier, help smooth day-to-day labor relations concerns, and help keep other bargaining units out of the organization.

UNEQUAL POSITIONS

Under the National Labor Relations Act, unions and employers do not have equal clout in the organizing process. In many respects the union enjoys the upper hand. Under the act an employer can commit a number of possible unfair labor practices and charges can be brought against the employer by the union. If the NLRB, ruling on an unfair labor practice charge, upholds the union's claim, then the union may be automatically certified as a recognized bargaining unit without a representation election.

The law, however, does not work in the opposite direction. Although there are a number of things that a union cannot legally do during organizing, for all practical purposes there is no such thing as an unfair labor practice committed by a union. Also, if the union should lose the election, it—or any other union seeking to represent the same employees—may petition for another election after one year has passed. The employer may well have to win year after year to remain nonunion. However, the employer need lose only once and the union is in, permanently for all practical purposes, because decertification of a union is difficult. (See the later section in this chapter concerning decertification.)

IF THE UNION WINS

Shortly after the union is certified as a recognized bargaining unit, an initial contract is negotiated. This gives managers an entirely new set of rules and regulations to live with.

The manager should learn the contract inside out—learn what it says, learn what it does not say, and learn why it says what it says—and comply with it faithfully. Some contracts may seem top-heavy with numerous details and exacting requirements, but some parts of the manager's job may actually be easier because there will now be hard-and-fast rules for some situations previously subject to interpretation and judgment.

The presence of a union, however, does not mean that the manager can back off in communications with employees and simply wave the contract at them. Complete two-way communication remains essential in establishing and maintaining relationships with all employees whether or not they are represented by a union. After all, the employees work for the institution, not for the union. Generally the union is the employees' voice only if the employees feel that they are not recognized as individuals and are not being heard by management.

DECERTIFICATION: REMOVING THE UNION

As compared with efforts to organize and obtain certification of a union as a collective bargaining agent, successful decertifications occur with dramatically lesser frequency. Also, many of the decertifications that do occur involve one union replacing another union, rather than removal of all union representation.

From its inception, the National Labor Relations Act has leaned strongly toward favoring unions and has built in a number of safeguards to protect employees from abuse by employers. In amending the NLRA, the 1947 Labor Management Reporting Act (known as the Taft-Hartley Act), took a more balanced approach in its efforts to protect the rights of employees from abuse by both employers and unions. Taft-Hartley permitted decertifications for the first time, making it possible for employees to get rid of a union they felt was not appropriately serving their purposes or acting in their best interests. Thanks to Taft-Hartley, employees could remove a union when they felt its leadership had failed to meet the expectations of the members or had failed to deliver on its preelection promises. Although permitted, decertifications are not especially common, but they do occur now and then.

A union's first year in place is referred to as the union's "certification year." A decertification petition cannot be filed within this initial year. A newly elected union is allowed this first year to negotiate a contract and show what it can do for those who voted it into power. Whether for initially choosing a union or attempting to decertify one, there can be only one representation election in a particular bargaining unit within a 12-month period.

Of primary importance to the department manager concerning decertification is that management is prohibited from any involvement in starting or encouraging a move toward decertification. Managers are not permitted to

- volunteer information about how employees can seek decertification;
- tell employees they would be better off without the union present (implied promises of improved treatment);
- encourage employees to start a decertification petition; or
- behave in any manner that could be construed as encouraging employees to pursue decertification.

For all practical purposes, all that management is legally allowed to do during the initiation of a decertification effort is to answer employees' questions about decertification. And this must be done without encouragement to pursue decertification and can include no unsolicited advice on how to go about doing so.

When decertification efforts reach the petition stage, the employer can still do little more than answer employees' questions. Now, however, that some responses can be more specific and therefore more helpful. For instance, management can tell employees how to contact the appropriate authorities at the NLRB and can provide additional information about the process as long as doing so is always in answer to employees' inquiries. However, this remains but minimal assistance considering that management is still not allowed to

- help write the petition, or allow the petition to be sent on the organization's official stationary;
- permit employees to collect petition signatures during working hours;
- provide management space for the petition signing; or
- provide time off for an employee to file the petition.

Once a decertification petition is filed and an election campaign officially starts, management has somewhat more freedom of participation subject to two important limitations: management may not interfere with the employees' right to choose between decertification or not, and management's behavior must be free from promises and threats and the like, which might be construed as affecting the conditions under which employees are to choose. During this process the "TIPS" rule is fully as applicable as during initial organizing. Management may express opinions about whether the union should remain or not, as long as these views carry no threats of reprisals for keeping the union or promises of rewards for removing the union. At this stage of the decertification campaign management is permitted to

- communicate its views and opinions to employees by letter;
- provide employees with comparisons of wages and benefits of union and nonunion workers; and
- meet with employees, providing employee attendance at such meetings is voluntary (that is, not mandated by management).

NOTES

1. M. Hudson, Unions Fight to Maintain Relevance, *Democrat and Chronicle*, Rochester, NY (September 2002).
2. Ibid.
3. Knight Ridder, Unions Set Sights on High-Tech Workers, *Democrat and Chronicle*, Rochester, NY (September 2000).

QUESTIONS AND ACTIVITIES

1. It is often claimed that many union elections are lost by management years before the organizers ever show up. Fully explain this statement.

2. Explain why, as stated in the text, it "could take 7 to 20 years to solve the nursing shortage."

3. List the advantages and disadvantages of having professional employees in the same union as nonprofessionals.

4. Imagine you are a working department manager. Fully explain to your employees where the money comes from to pay the union's external organizers and support the local union's officers.

5. State the strongest case you can make *in favor* of unions for professional employees.

6. State the strongest case you can make *in opposition* to unions for professional employees.

QUESTIONS AND ACTIVITIES *(continued)*

7. Your organization is experiencing active union organizing. A loyal, long-time employee in your department asks you if you would like her to attend this weekend's scheduled union meeting and report back to you. What will you tell her, and why?

8. List the advantages and disadvantages of having as many as eight bargaining units within the same organization, and decide if overall this condition is desirable or undesirable.

9. Take a position either in favor or against having first-line managers in the same union as their employees. (This is frequently the case in governmental health care institutions that have public employee unions.) Justify your position.

10. Concerning an organization's vulnerability to union organizing, explain why it could be especially important to professional employees for there to be the opportunity for input to organizational processes.

11. One of your better employees asks what you think about the union that is attempting to organize at your institution. Explain how you will answer this question.

12. Although management is legally prohibited from making promises to employees to get them to reject a union, the union may make all the promises it wishes to induce the employees to accept the union. Explain why this seeming contradiction exists.

13. An employee tells you that he signed a union authorization card, but that he now has second thoughts. He wants to know how to get the card back or have it withdrawn. What can you tell him?

14. Many employees claim that they organize in search of respect and other intangibles, but when a union enters into contract negotiations almost everything demanded has a monetary cost attached to it. Why do you believe this is so?

15. One of your employees asks you directly, "Why don't you want us to join a union?" How will you answer?

16. Explain why a first-line or middle manager might be sympathetic to the employees' desire for a union, and might thus passively support the union's organizing efforts.

QUESTIONS AND ACTIVITIES *(continued)*

17. Often a union interested in organizing in a specific institution will work quietly and well undercover for some time before its organizers reveal their presence. Explain why you believe this particular strategy is employed.

18. On the way to a meeting that is about to begin, you are accosted in a busy hospital corridor by three of your employees. One of them says to you, "It's about time we learned where you stand on this union thing. We need to talk—right now." How are you going to respond?

19. Fully explain what you believe a union that represents your employees must do to maintain its perceived usefulness to the employees.

20. You are walking through one of the hospital's departments during normal working hours when you see a service employee backed into a corner by a person who is waving in the employee's face what appears to be a union authorization card. Explain what you would do (a) if you think you recognize the apparent organizer as an employee; and (b) if you feel certain the organizer is not an employee of the hospital.

CHAPTER 12

Cases: Managing the Health Care Professional

Never cut what you can untie.
—Joseph Joubert

If anything can happen, it will.
—Murphy

This Chapter Will:

▶ Provide the reader with the opportunity to consider the contents of the preceding chapters as they apply to case studies based on problems and situations taken from actual work settings.

USE OF THE CASE STUDIES

Case studies represent an extremely useful means of testing one's knowledge and judgment. They also provide an opportunity for one to consider how particular principles and techniques might be applied in real-world situations. When going through any collection of cases, though, one may quickly form the impression that there are few absolute, specific answers to the problems posed and the situations presented. For this reason this chapter does not include specific answers to the cases presented, because so few absolute answers are possible. Some problems may be solved in several different ways—all of them in their own way appropriate—depending on differences among the people involved and differences in organization policy, philosophy of operation, and the environment in which the situations occur. Most of the cases concern the interrelationships among people; this should come as no surprise because the essence of management consists of getting things done through people. We can of course postulate some rules for dealing with people—for instance, we can surely agree that all employees are deserving of fair and equal treatment—but most of the less generalized "rules" we might cite would be riddled with exceptions.

In some of the cases presented in this chapter, certain management fundamentals or basic principles, such as fair and equal treatment of employees, might be self-evident. However, many supposed solutions to case studies take forms such as, "What might happen if I do this?" or "I'll take this action, and if this particular result occurs I'll then proceed to try this other remedy." Or simply: "This might work, or at least it seems fair and it makes sense."

It should be evident to most working managers that there are few guaranteed solutions to their problems. Frustrating as it seems, the correct solution to a given problem involving one employee might not be correct should a different employee be involved. If one has a dozen employees in a group, one may find that on any given day there can be as many as 12 "right" ways of dealing with employees on a particular issue. Managers should certainly strive to be consistent in their application of principles and in their treatment of employees as individuals. However, the employees of a department are likely to be anything but consistent in their response to the manager's actions.

Case studies help narrow the gap between theory and practice. However, in matters of actual practice a case is just a simulation. Although a case may be *based* on a real problem, it is not itself a real problem because it no longer involves real people in the here and now, and in particular it lacks the emotional involvement that a manager experiences with a real problem. Nevertheless, the case study represents a giant step away from theory and toward matters of practice. A primary purpose of the case method is to encourage the development and exploration of alternatives. The principal benefits of the case study method lie not in the identification of answers but in the development of insights.

This chapter includes 21 cases: One fully developed example, plus 20 additional cases for reader consideration. These cases are described by a topic emphasis—the principal topic of the case—and by the enumeration of two, three, or four additional topics for which the case provides food for thought.

A CASE STUDY EXAMPLE

A fully developed example is provided in the form of a case and a compilation of a number of potential responses to the situation described in the case. In developing the responses, effort was made to come as close as practical to exhausting all significant avenues of consideration. As a result, the responses presented herein are likely to be considerably longer and more detailed than any single workable approach might be. Thus the responses include the bases for several potentially productive ways of approaching the problem, any of which might or might not work depending on the personalities involved.

EXAMPLE CASE

Topic emphasis: Communication

Additional topics: Criticism and discipline

People problems

"HAVE YOU EVER ONCE BEEN WRONG?"

"There's no doubt about what I heard, just a few simple words in plain English," snapped staff nurse Beth Miller. Beth's expression was dark and she spoke in that sternly righteous tone that nurse manager Carrie Summer had heard so many times before.

"That's not what Dr. Parker says, Beth," said Carrie. "He told me quite specifically that he gave you simple, clear instructions but you went and did exactly the opposite of what he ordered. And he really came on strongly."

"Tough," said Beth. "He's wrong."

"He says that you were the one who was wrong, and he seemed quite certain of his position. He explained the entire situation to me, and I have to admit that I understood his instructions right away. At least I was able to repeat what he said in my own words so that he was satisfied I understood what he told me."

Beth shook her head, then shrugged and said, "So Parker changed his story between the time we talked and the time he spoke with you. Par for the course around here."

"Are you saying that Dr. Parker lied to me?"

"I didn't say, one way or the other. I'm only saying that he told me one thing and then apparently told you something else. Maybe he didn't realize what he was saying to one or the other of us. Or maybe he realizes he made a mistake and is trying to dump it off on me. Anyway, you know how he just spouts off something on the run and doesn't stay around to find out if he's been understood."

Carrie sighed and said, "Beth, did you consider the possibility that *you* didn't understand? It's pretty easy to misinterpret a message when things are happening as fast as they do around here."

Beth snapped, "I know what I heard. When I know I'm wrong, I'll say so. If there's even a possibility that I'm wrong, I'll admit to it. But in this case I know I'm right. It's not even remotely likely that I misinterpreted what Dr. Parker told me."

Carrie felt that there had been too many times in their relationship that Beth had come across in this completely inflexible manner. She also felt that via her attitude Beth had provided reason for Carrie to speak up about something that had been nagging at her for nearly as long as she and Beth had worked together. Making no effort to hide her exasperation, Carrie said, "Beth, have you ever once been wrong?"

Beth glared at her manager. "And just what is that supposed to mean?"

Carrie paused for a deep breath, then said, "Beth, I've been nurse manager of this unit for going on three years, and in all that time I've never known you to admit to being wrong about anything. This issue with Dr. Parker is just one more example of how you always turn things around so that you look innocent or correct. Is it so necessary that you be right about everything?"

Beth's tone, already cool, became colder still. "I already said that I'll admit I'm wrong, but only when I really am wrong. And I want to know the other times you're talking about, the times when I supposedly turned things around as you claim I did."

Carrie said, "Well, there was—." She stopped, frowned and shook her head, and continued. "No, I was thinking about something else. In any case, you ought to know what I'm talking about. Think about it and you'll know what I mean. You always have an answer for everything, and it's always the answer that makes you right and everyone else wrong."

Beth snapped, "You can't think of any specific incidents because there haven't been any. The only problem here is that you don't particularly like me." She rose from her chair and moved a step toward the door. "You may be my immediate supervisor, but I don't have to listen to your accusations. Is there anything else you want to say about *Dr. Parker's* problem?" She glared at Carrie.

Carrie rose to her feet. "Just that the incident is not to be considered closed. Dr. Parker insists that it be written up for disciplinary action, at least a first-step warning."

Beth said, "I'll fight it, of course. I won't accept a warning that I don't deserve, and I won't say I was wrong when I know I was right."

When Beth had left the office, Carrie began to regret having spoken as she did. She was convinced, however, that she had to try to get through to Beth about her apparent need to be right whenever a disagreement or misunderstanding arose.

Questions:

1. When Carrie abandoned the specific incident to talk about Beth's overall behavior, she made a mistake that is embodied in her words: "—you

always turn things around so that you look innocent or correct." What was the mistake, and why was it a mistake?

2. How would you recommend attempting to determine the cause of the misunderstanding involving Beth and Dr. Parker?

3. Taking Beth's unhappy departure from Carrie's office as your starting point, how would you propose to deal with an employee who seems unable to admit to ever being wrong?

Responses:

Question #1

There were actually two errors, one implicit in the comments preceding Carrie's statement and one explicit in the statement itself. The implicit error lies in Carrie's surrender to an emotional reaction. The explicit error was Carrie's abandonment of a specific issue for the sake of generalization.

It is understandable for Carrie to act emotionally regarding a longstanding problem that had been "nagging at her" for some time. However, the fact of her giving voice to her accumulated frustrations at this particular time when she is attempting to resolve a specific difficulty serves only to destroy the focus of the discussion. Carrie may not be able to help experiencing an emotional reaction, but an outward exhibition of that emotional reaction does not take her any closer to a solution for the specific problem. In fact, in most cases such a reaction takes the parties to the discussion in opposite directions, away from resolution of the problem. The situation suggests that Carrie allowed a number of past problems and continuing frustrations to take over and channel her comments in unproductive directions.

In one-to-one communication it is almost invariably true that the opportunity for meaningful dialogue is diminished as emotion intrudes into the discussion. In this instance, Carrie's reaction was voiced in a blanket condemnation of Beth's communication tendencies, and in doing so Carrie openly invited an emotional response from Beth.

Carrie was incorrect in abandoning the specific issue and resorting to generality, especially without proof of any wrongdoing beyond that concerned with the specific incident involving Dr. Parker. Rather, she should have remained limited to the specific item under discussion. In telling Beth that she is projecting a supposed attitude of never being wrong, Carrie is giving Beth reason to believe that her word is constantly being doubted.

Carrie appears to have lost sight of one of the fundamental rules of one-to-one communication: Whenever possible, leave the other party some maneuvering space by leaving some options open, or by making it clear that there is always room for reasonable doubt. The key word in Carrie's statement is *always*, as in "you always turn things around so you look innocent or correct." The party who says, "You always do this" is, first, making a statement that is rarely true in an absolute sense because *always* is an all-inclusive term. Second, they are putting the other party into a corner from which there is no face-saving exit. Carrie put Beth in a corner, and Beth reacted as one might expect any person to react when cornered—defensively.

When cornered, Beth's defensive reaction was to immediately challenge her attacker. She reacted, quite reasonably so, by asking for specific incidents: the other times when she supposedly turned things around. Because Carrie did not have the recollection of any previous specific incidents close at hand, her response was extremely weak and she instantly found herself on the defensive; she continued to criticize Beth in general terms. This is the way that any two-person interchange is likely to go when emotion has taken over and general charges of wrongdoing are resorted to; the conversation falls into a pattern of alternating attack and defense from which neither participant can derive a satisfactory solution.

Were Carrie to have strayed from the specific problem and opened up the discussion to include broader criticism of Beth's conduct, she should have done so only if she could use specific incidents of a similar nature for which hard evidence or past resolution was available.

Question #2

It would be desirable to get the disagreeing parties, Beth and Dr. Parker, together for a discussion of the present difficulty. In doing so Carrie should make every effort to avoid clearly taking sides in the matter or even projecting the notion that she might be taking sides. If in the absence of any clear immediate proof that favors one party over the other Carrie exhibits any leaning at all, it should be in the direction of her employee, Beth. Employees need to be able to count on their manager's backing when conflicts occur with persons outside the department, and a certain measure of Carrie's support was due Beth if only on the basis of innocence until proven guilty. Carrie should be especially mindful of the temptation to defer to the power of a physician without giving the employee a fair hearing.

If the conflict involves a practice for which orders or instructions are customarily written, Carrie would need to reinforce with both parties the necessity to commit certain requests to writing. In addition to being required by various accrediting and regulatory bodies, written orders and instructions tend to protect the best interests of both parties. They also provide a permanent record that reduces the chance of misunderstanding.

Regardless of the righteous posture of either party to the dispute, Carrie should assume that an equal chance for misunderstanding exists with each. If there is nothing in writing, and as long as the dispute remains in the realm of one's word against another's, Carrie should attempt to sell both parties on a no-penalty solution. Beth may have to be convinced that she needs to concede to Dr. Parker and assure that something is done his way. However, Dr. Parker probably has to be convinced that even though he stands as "right," there should be no official warning because a warning based on hearsay is not valid.

If a third party witnessed the original contact between Beth and Dr. Parker, Carrie should consider seeking out the third party and comparing that person's version of what happened with the claims of the participants in the dispute. Carrie has gotten into deeper difficulty because she projected a bias based on past problems with Beth; however, it might be equally as likely that Dr. Parker also has generated a history of communication problems. Knowledge of such recurring problems might be helpful to Carrie in deciding how to approach the participants in the disagreement.

Carrie's role should be that of diplomat and peacemaker in this situation. She should attempt to minimize hard feelings resulting from the incident and find ways to help the parties reach agreement so that all may get back to the business of patient care. Finding someone to blame should not be her concern; she should be seeking to solve the problem, not trying to assign blame.

Question #3

The key to Carrie's future dealings with the employee who seems to believe she is never wrong is to deal only with specific instances and rely heavily on documentation. If Beth's conduct is called into question but the specific incident is not provable, Carrie should let the incident go as though it had never happened and save her energies for dealings in which she is able to offer proof. If Beth is indeed the kind of person who absolutely must be right, it is doubtful that anything that Carrie ever does would inspire basic change in Beth's character. One occasionally encounters people for whom communication is always a win-or-lose proposition; when they win they are "right" and when they lose they are "wrong." These people do not like to lose and are often incapable of admitting a loss.

There are some additional pointers for Carrie to keep in mind in future dealings with Beth:

- Reinforce the use, whenever practical, of written orders and instructions as opposed to those transmitted orally.

- In face-to-face dealings with Beth, conduct conversations in such a way that true two-way interchange is necessary. When giving an order or instruction, Carrie should put it in such a way that Beth must repeat the message in her own words so that both parties can agree on what was said.

In general, Carrie must avoid using the words *always* and *never*, which increase the likelihood of leaving Beth, or any other party, no escape from the situation. She must always leave room for negotiation and compromise.

On occasions when Beth is indeed right, let her know that she is right. If Beth is to hear about her errors, she should also hear about her successes.

If it becomes necessary to apply the progressive disciplinary process (an oral warning and other steps that follow in order of seriousness), Carrie should take great pains to ensure that Beth has numerous opportunities along the way to correct the behavior problem. Keep in mind that in the majority of cases, the true purpose of the disciplinary process is not to punish but rather to correct or improve behavior.

THE CASES

CASE 1

Topic emphasis:	Change management
Additional topics:	People problems
	Leadership

CAROL'S CHOICE

When nurse manager Carol Summer was faced with the task of promoting one of her full-time staff members to the position of assistant nurse manager, she found that she did not lack for qualified employees. There was considerable longevity and experience represented in her unit, and it seemed to her that the real task might not be deciding who could do the job but rather deciding which of the several people who apparently wanted the job should be bypassed. After thinking her way through a number of possible choices, Carol narrowed the field to two people that she felt were equally outstanding candidates. Jane West and Helen Wright, who Carol felt were probably the two best nurses in the unit, appeared equal to each other in qualifications and experience in just about every aspect.

It was clear to Carol that both Jane and Helen wanted the assistant nurse manager position. Each had made her desires known to Carol upon first learning that the position was opening up. Both Jane and Helen were relatively energetic and appeared to be career-oriented.

Carol made her choice, and with the blessing of nursing administration she promoted Jane West to assistant nurse manager. Although she did not discuss the reasons for her decision with anyone, Carol admitted to herself that her decision was based largely on personality; Jane seemed friendlier than Helen, and more able to relate to other people on a one-to-one basis.

Jane eagerly accepted the promotion and plunged into her new role with enthusiasm. Helen expressed some initial disappointment, which seemed at least to Carol to dissipate fairly quickly.

However, six weeks after Jane's promotion it was plain to Carol that Helen had changed both her outlook and her behavior. Where Helen had once always seemed ready and willing to do her share of work and then some, she now seemed satisfied doing just enough to get by. Although never overly talkative or socially outgoing, Helen seemed to become silent and withdrawn. Worst of all, at least to Carol, was Helen's apparent practice of resisting instructions from the new assistant nurse manager and creating obstacles for Jane.

Carol realized that she had a problem that required her active involvement when she overheard Helen grumbling about how "a person has to be the nurse manager's buddy to get anywhere around here."

Questions:

1. How might unintended personal bias have intruded into Carol's selection of Jane over Helen?

2. What do events after Jane's promotion say about Carol's choice of a charge nurse?

3. How should Carol deal with Helen?

CASE 2

Topic emphasis:	Delegation
Additional topics:	Management style
	Leadership

THE DUAL ROLE:
SHOULD THE MANAGER DO NONMANAGEMENT WORK?

Susan James served as administrative manager of the department of diagnostic imaging. She was a classic example of a manager who came up through the ranks: She had been chief technologist for the department, a special procedures technician, a member of the larger technician group handling routine procedures, and, years earlier, a student at the hospital's school of radiologic technology.

Susan had an impressive background in special procedures and had acquired considerable academic and technical knowledge in radiation safety. As a result, in the two years since becoming department manager she had been called upon increasingly often to substitute for the radiation safety officer in important technical matters, and also to fill in as a special procedures technician. More and more, however, she found herself resisting technical intrusions on her management role to a point at which it became evident that Dr. Grainger, the chief of diagnostic imaging, was growing impatient with her.

One day at a special meeting she was asked by her manager, the vice president for ancillary services, "What's happened between you and Dr. Grainger? He says you seemed to be put out when you were asked to fill in for special procedures, and he also suggested that the last couple of meetings of the radiation safety committee pretty much fell apart because you were unwilling to take the chair and see that things got done. Do you feel that something's changing for the worse? Perhaps your work is piling up to where it's no longer controllable?"

Susan shook her head impatiently. "'No, it's not that. I think my workload is well under control. And I know that radiation safety needs help because of Harriet's recurring problems, and the turnover in special procedures is killing us because those people are in such short supply in this area. What I think the problem really is—I don't think I'm comfortable in the dual role, mainly because I don't know if what seems to be expected of me is right for me to be doing as a manager."

"Meaning what?"

"Meaning, am I a manager or am I a technical person? I think I know special procedures and radiation safety fairly well. But it doesn't take a manager to serve as radiation safety officer, and, if I allowed it to do so, radiation safety could take so much of my time that department management would really suffer. And I'm not sure that I belong in special procedures any longer."

The vice president for ancillary services asked, "Why do you say that? You were one of the best special procedures techs this place ever had."

"I like to think so, but times change and it's been a long time since I've done that day in and day out. More than half the equipment in those rooms has changed since I worked there full time. One of the last times I was in there at Dr. Grainger's request one of the special procedures techs—the only full-time tech we have left in that area—said he'd rather not have my help because coaching me along would slow him down and he could do it faster without me. Plus the last time I helped out with routine procedures during a crunch one of the techs made a comment about me 'slumming.' Someone else even suggested that I was there simply to 'see how the other half lives.'"

After a moment Susan concluded, "I've always believed that the basic job of a manager was to get things done through people, and I've tried to practice that as long as I've been in management. I guess I'm afraid that doing all of this technical work is somehow making me less of a manager."

Questions:

1. Do you agree that the performance of the technical work as described is making Susan less of a manager, as she fears? Explain your answer.

2. Given that delegation is one of a manager's most important activities, identify and describe: one set of conditions or circumstances under which Susan's involvement in the technical tasks described is fully appropriate, and one set of conditions or circumstances under which Susan's technical-task involvement would be inappropriate.

CASE 3

Topic emphasis:	Professional behavior
Additional topics:	Communication
	Leadership
	Management Style
	Authority

A MEETING OF PROFESSIONALS?

There are 15 people in your department, about two-thirds of whom are health care professionals. It has been a long-standing practice in the department, going well back before your time as manager, to convene a staff meeting at 3:00 P.M.

every Wednesday. Rather, we should say that you *attempt* to convene the meeting at 3:00 because about half of your employees are 5 to 10 minutes late and two or three others are usually late by 15 minutes or longer. Nearly all of the consistently tardy attendees are professionals.

You have made repeated announcements about being there on time but these seem to have had no effect. When 3:00 P.M. Wednesday arrives, you usually find yourself and the same six or seven punctual attendees—including all but one of the department's few nonprofessionals—present and waiting for the latecomers.

Of those who consistently arrive late, a few take the trouble to offer reasons why they could not be there on time. However, several of the professionals offer no reasons or excuses for their tardiness, and the attitude, behavior, and lack of active participation of some of them suggests they would just as soon not be there at all.

Question:

Without immediately considering disciplinary action (which with all employees, professional and otherwise, should always be the last resort following consideration of all reasonable alternatives), what can you do to encourage punctuality for employees attending your staff meetings?

CASE 4

Topic emphasis:	Delegation
Additional topics:	Communication
	Professional behavior
	Motivation
	Management style

"I'M ONLY DOING WHAT I'M TOLD TO DO"

The health information management (HIM) department of the 600-bed Memorial Hospital was considered, when necessary, able to function for a week or so at a time without its director. Each of the two significant divisions of the department was headed by a registered record administrator (R.R.A.), so someone possessing the appropriate credentials was always available. However, when Mrs. Johnson, director of HIM, was hospitalized for several weeks, Mrs. Johnson's immediate superior, vice president George Smith, began to take an active interest in the daily management of HIM to the extent of at least monitoring what the two division managers were doing.

At about noon one day, George noticed a completed form entitled "Daily Census Report" on the corner of the desk of one of the HIM division managers. It caught his eye because in his few months at Memorial Hospital the only census report he had seen was the computer-generated report he received each morning. He became even more curious when he noticed that the apparently hand-compiled report bore this day's date. He asked the manager, Carol Wilson, who created the report and why it was done.

"Sometimes I do it, and sometimes Angela prepares it" she said, nodding toward the desk of one of the clerical staff, "but I don't really know why it's done." She proceeded to describe the process: Each morning the previous day's HIM count of admissions and discharges was merged with the information obtained from the midnight census report generated by nursing. This took either Carol or Angela about an hour and a half each day.

George asked, "Who uses this report?"

"I don't think anybody uses it."

"Then let me put it this way," said George, frustration mounting, "who gets the report?"

"Nobody," Carol answered. She went on to explain that some time earlier there were problems occurring with a computer system changeover and certain census information was being lost. Her manager, Mrs. Johnson, showed her how to do the report and told her where to leave it. For two or three weeks the report was picked up at noon every day.

"Why hasn't it been discontinued?" asked George.

"It was discontinued once," Carol answered. "By me. And I got into plenty of trouble over it. It got picked up regularly for a while, but someone stopped coming for it and before I knew it I had eight or nine on my desk. I tried to ask Mrs. Johnson about it but I still couldn't get an answer—you can never get her to stand still for 10 seconds—so I just stopped doing it on my own because I couldn't see any sense in it. When Mrs. Johnson found out I dropped it she gave me the chewing out of my life and said that I'd better never do anything like that again without a direct order. That was months ago."

George asked, "Haven't you tried to bring it up again?"

"Yes, but I don't think it ever sank in. She's always busy, always in a hurry, and the only people who seem able to get her attention for more than a minute at a time are administration and the doctors. Once she said she'd look into it, but I haven't heard anything. And I'm not sticking my neck out again. I'm only doing what I'm told to do."

George spent a few more minutes with Carol looking over some of the reports. In that time he discovered that both Carol and Angela had done neat, accurate work, taking as long as 90 minutes a day, for longer than a year. And 11 months worth of this work resided in a file drawer in HIM, never seen by anyone other than Carol and Angela.

Questions:

1. Who do you believe is responsible for the duration of this apparently unnecessary task? Why?

2. Describe the fundamental errors that appear to have caused the perpetuation of the manually generated report.

3. What should George do with his newly acquired information?

4. Comment at whatever length you believe necessary on the attitude and behavior of Carol.

CASE 5

Topic emphasis:	Management style
Additional topics:	Communication
	Professional behavior
	Employee relations

THE D. I.

One day while shopping in a local market, Donna Roberts, nurse manager of one of the larger medical/surgical units at County Hospital, encountered Regina Trent, a neighbor and acquaintance and also one of the registered nurses in Donna's unit. After a bit of small talk Donna said to Regina, "I know that since you went part-time you've been working every other weekend. Elaine Bliss, our new weekend charge nurse, came in about the same time you changed over. How is it going working with her?"

After some hesitation Regina said, "Honestly, Donna—and this is just between the two of us, after hours and away from the hospital—I don't like working for her at all."

A somewhat surprised Donna countered, "May I ask why?"

"To me her entire approach, her manner with all of the staff, is inappropriate," said Regina. "She's curt and snappish. She never asks people to do things, she just barks orders. She usually sounds more like an army sergeant than a charge nurse. In fact, thanks to Karl Gross—the new R.N. who came to us from the Army Nurse Corps—a number of the staff now refer to her as the D. I."

"D. I.?"

"Drill instructor. And a couple of the others have said that working is anything but bliss when Bliss in is charge."

Although Donna realized she was hearing but a single person's view, she was disturbed by this informal report on a weekend charge nurse whom she had appointed. It was true that Elaine appeared no more or less qualified than a number of other available nurses, but Elaine had no objection to working weekends and had seemed to Donna even to welcome the opportunity. For three days each week, Elaine was simply one of the capable nurses on the unit. However, Donna had to admit that she knew nothing about how Elaine was working out as weekend charge because she had never seen her in action in that capacity. Until her conversation with Regina, Donna had received no reports about Elaine's behavior.

Even though the need to do Elaine's first performance appraisal as weekend charge nurse was months away, Donna decided she had best look into the matter of Elaine's performance immediately. Over the next two weeks Donna sought out most of her unit's weekend workers for individual discussions. In each discussion she was no more specific in her initial questioning than, "How are you getting along with our new weekend charge?" However, this approach was sufficient: Donna had known most of the staff for several years, and the majority of them were willing to speak freely and did so with no additional encouragement from Donna.

In the process of her one-on-one meetings, Donna learned that several weekend staff believed that Elaine's authoritarian approach was directly responsible for the resignation of one nurse who cited "personal reasons" for leaving. During her discussions Donna also heard the following comments about Elaine:

- "During the week when she's not in charge she's okay to work with, but on the weekends she's a terror."

- "She orders us around like a drill sergeant."

- "She doesn't do much herself, just tells everybody else what to do."

- "I think being in charge has gone to her head. She really likes to lord it over everyone."

Overall, Donna was quite discouraged by all the second-hand information she had acquired about the style of her weekend charge nurse, Elaine.

Question:

How do you believe Donna should proceed in addressing the problems apparently presented by the weekend charge nurse? Outline your steps or options, and supply a complete rationale or justification for each.

CASE 6

Topic emphasis:	Communication
Additional topics:	Professional behavior
	Leadership
	Motivation
	Management style

THE SILENCER

James Argus, a management consultant specializing in health care matters, was engaged by the board of directors of a small rural hospital to study communication within the organization and to assess employee attitude. He was to focus especially on the attitudes and communications effectiveness of supervisors and managers.

James arranged to hold informal discussion meetings, essentially "rap sessions," with the entire management group each Monday. So as not to disrupt operations more than necessary, it was arranged for Argus to meet with half of the management group from 8:30 A.M. to 10:00 A.M. and the other half from 10:30 A.M. until noon. He was to do this each week for several weeks, while visiting the facility on other occasions to study organization structure, reporting relationships, and various aspects of departmental activity. The facility's chief executive officer told James in advance that he doubted the sessions would accomplish much; his management group consisted mostly of "close-mouthed people" who opened up only with great difficulty. James had to understand, said the CEO, that this facility was the largest employer in a small, isolated community, and that few people here would be likely to speak freely with "an outsider," especially in the presence of their peers. Thus forewarned, James launched his first Monday session with some discussion-oriented case material which he hoped would get people talking.

On the first two Mondays James felt as though he may as well have been alone in the room. Each group was as silent as the other. The only comments offered were strictly related to the case material he had brought along; he could get no one to acknowledge any connection with conditions at the hospital.

On the first two Mondays the CEO attended the earlier session, as did a dozen or so other people of varying management levels, including the hospital's second-in-command who served in the dual capacity of assistant administrator and personnel director.

However, the CEO was absent from the third early session, and James finally managed to create an opening in the wall that had confronted him. Evidently encouraged by something brought up in the course of a case discussion, one supervisor began to relate a problem based on an incident that had apparently left him in a bad light in the eyes of his employees, and had caused embarrassment for two other supervisors. Although the supervisor mentioned no names, the story's disguise was sufficiently thin for the several participants—and their errors—to be recognizable. The discussion, however, was rational, if somewhat spirited, and a number of people made favorable comments to James after the session was over.

The people in the late morning session also opened up, fully as enthusiastic as the ones in the earlier group. James could only guess that a few comments had been exchanged between sessions.

When James arrived for the fourth Monday's early session he was greeted by dead silence and long faces. There were several latecomers, and he noted several absences. The assistant administrator was there, but the CEO was absent. The late morning group was fully as silent as the earlier group, and there was one change in the composition of the group—the CEO was now a participant. Now the facility's top managers were divided, with one of them in each session.

For the rest of the series of sessions the assistant administrator remained with the early group and the CEO stayed with the later group. After the seventh scheduled session James called a halt to the series. Four straight sessions had produced little more than silence, which, along with facial expressions and other body language told him a great deal about the state of the organization.

Questions:

1. Explain what you believe is likely to have caused both groups to revert to silence after "opening up" during the third session.

2. Explain in detail what James might have been able to infer from the behavior of the two discussion groups.

CASE 7

Topic emphasis:	Professional behavior
Additional topics:	Employee relations
	Motivation
	People problems

THE BULLY

Wende Carlson, office manager for the hospital's ambulatory services division, was secretly happy that her half-day conference had been in the morning and not in the afternoon. Mornings in the office were so frantic and stressful that Wende was more than happy to miss a morning once in a while. Afternoons were relatively quiet, so Wende had hopes of getting caught up on some delinquent paperwork after returning from her outside commitment. However, when she arrived at her office after lunch, she was greeted by four angry expressions and one empty desk.

Indicating the empty desk, Wende asked, "Where's Sue? And why the stone faces? What's going on around here?"

"Sue went home," Eleanor said.

"She had to go home after Dr. Greer got through with her," said Kay. "I think I would've spit in his eye and walked out for good."

Wende asked, "What in the world happened?"

Eleanor explained, "Sue had the misfortune to make a simple booking mistake when Dr. Greer was at his busiest. He's a bear most of the time anyway, and we all know how he's been lately with the group running one physician short."

Wende said, "We obviously shouldn't make booking errors, but as hectic as it gets around here they're bound to happen once in a while and there's usually nothing serious about them."

Kay said, "You'd think they were life-threatening the way he took off on her. He called her about 10 different kinds of an idiot and said he was going to have her fired for incompetence. He literally screamed at her, in front of the four of us and Dr. Wilson and at least three or four patients in the waiting area."

"No class, rotten style," Eleanor muttered. The others nodded in agreement. "Why did Sue go home?" Wende asked.

Eleanor answered, "Greer really leveled her and ordered her out of the office. She cried in the ladies room for nearly half an hour, but even after she calmed down a bit she was afraid to come back in. She just signed out and went home."

In further discussion with her four staff members, Wende learned that Sue had stated there was no way she could continue working where she was treated in that fashion and that Dr. Greer had announced for all to hear that she was forbidden ever to touch his schedules again.

Questions:

1. Assume you are in Wende's position and describe how you would approach the discussion of the incident with Sue.

2. Recognizing that Dr. Greer is neither her employer nor her organizational superior, describe how you believe Wende should approach discussion of the incident with Dr. Greer.

3. Outline the steps you believe Wende should consider in addressing the problem presented by "The Bully," and in attempting to repair the apparent damage caused within her work group. Provide detailed reasons for your recommendations.

CASE 8

Topic emphasis:	Criticism and discipline
Additional topics:	Professional behavior
	Motivation
	Communication
	People problems

THE DODGER

June Watson had considerable difficulty developing the schedule for her nursing unit for the coming two weeks. The nursing department was in a marginal position overall as far as staffing was concerned, so her flexibility was limited. To make matters worse, within hours after June issued the newest schedule Alice Jackson, a part-time registered nurse, submitted a request for a personal day on one of the days she was scheduled to work.

The request caused June to realize that she had been seeing Alice's name in connection with scheduling difficulties often in recent months. Looking back over the preceding six months' worth of schedules she discovered that the current request made the fifth time in six months that Alice had requested time off on a scheduled weekend day. Even more significant was the pattern of Alice's use of sick time. She had called in sick four times, all of these on Saturdays or Sundays. All in all, Alice had worked only about half of the weekend days she had been scheduled to work over a period of six months.

June was displeased with Alice's attendance and unhappy with herself for not discovering the problem sooner. She felt she had to talk with Alice about it, but she also felt that her unit could ill afford to lose a nurse. Staffing had been so tight that many of the nurse managers were putting up with a certain amount of inappropriate behavior simply to avoid risking the loss of nurses and worsening their staffing situation. Nevertheless, June believed that she could not allow Alice's attendance practices to continue uncorrected.

Questions:

1. Describe in detail the hazards that June may face in (a) dealing firmly and directly with Alice's behavior, and (b) ignoring Alice's absences and saying nothing.

2. Assuming June is planning on talking with Alice about her attendance, describe how she might most constructively approach the problem and identify alternative approaches that might be considered depending on Alice's reaction and response.

CASE 9

Topic emphasis:	Management authority
Additional topics:	Professional behavior
	Hiring and firing
	Relations with superiors
	Criticism and correction

HE DIDN'T WORK OUT

Bill Young, a graduate mechanical engineer, was hired by James Memorial Hospital as manager of plant engineering and maintenance. Although he had 15 years experience in the field this was Bill's first management position.

Shortly after Bill's arrival, a maintenance helper job became available. This was an important job because of the numerous preventive maintenance tasks involved, and Bill recognized the need to fill this position as soon as possible. Immediately after receiving the departing helper's resignation, Bill asked the human resources department to locate several candidates for him to interview.

Bill's immediate supervisor, chief operating officer Peter Jackson, chose to sit in on the interviews, giving as his reason Bill's newness to management. Peter indicated that because Bill had never interviewed or hired before, he should be assisted in the process.

Bill and Peter jointly interviewed five candidates. Of the five, two appeared to be reasonably qualified for the job. One of these was a young man named Simmons, who was employed in the hospital's food service department. The other was a young man named Kelly who had not worked recently but had several months of building-and-grounds experience at a school.

Following the interviews, Bill expressed his desired to hire Simmons from food service because he appeared to have the aptitude and ability and exhibited a strong desire to better himself. Bill also reasoned that selecting Simmons would show that the hospital was genuinely interested in developing employees within the organization. However, Peter disagreed and told Bill he could do the hiring "the next time a job opened." Peter himself made the decision to hire Kelly and personally communicated the offer to Kelly.

As the 30-day probationary period progressed it became increasingly evident to Bill that Kelly was not shaping up as a satisfactory employee. Even while being certain to give Kelly all reasonable orientation and guidance, and extending every benefit of the doubt because he had been "the boss's choice," Bill could conclude only that they would be making a mistake keeping Kelly on past the introductory period.

On the twenty-eighth day of Kelly's employment Bill went to see Peter. He had kept Peter advised of Kelly's poor progress and lack of response to guidance, so it was no surprise to Peter when Bill said they should let Kelly go and start all over again.

"Okay," Peter replied, "let Kelly go."

Bill hesitated, wondering a moment if he should say anything, and finally said to Peter, "I don't believe I should be the one to let him go. I'm not the one who hired him."

"He's your employee," Peter responded. "You get rid of him."

Questions:

1. Do you believe Peter was correct in ordering Bill to discharge Kelly, or do you feel that he simply dodged responsibility by doing so? Be thorough in providing reasons for your response.

2. Describe at least two additional ways in which this situation could have been more equitably handled.

3. Explain what effects the Kelly incident could have on the future relationship between Bill and Peter.

CASE 10

Topic emphasis:	People problems
Additional topics:	Professional behavior
	Interpersonal relations
	Management authority

THE DEPARTMENT'S RESIDENT "EXPERT"

Several weeks ago physical therapist Walt Palmer said to his manager, director of physical therapy George Jackson, "You know, George, the way we go about developing the budget in this department doesn't make a whole lot of sense. All we do is take last year's actual expenses and add on an inflation factor and make some other guesses. What we really ought to be doing is budgeting from a zero base, making every line item completely justify itself every year."

George said something about simply following the budgeting instructions issued by the finance department and doing it the way he was told. He pursued the matter no further.

A few days following the budget question, Walt approached George with another suggestion: "Don't you think the way we do performance appraisals ought to change? Most smart managers know it's better to evaluate employees on their anniversary dates than the way we do it, trying to evaluate everyone during the same short stretch of time."

George again answered to the effect that as a manager he was simply doing what he had to do to comply with the policies and practices of the organization. They discussed the matter for perhaps five minutes, and although George was not about to start working to stimulate change in the performance appraisal system, he nevertheless felt that Walt had brought up a number of good points. It struck George that his employee was idealizing an evaluation system in textbook terms; it seemed flawless in theory, but George had been through enough actual systems to be able to recognize a number of potential barriers to thorough practical application of what Walt was suggesting.

In the ensuing two to three weeks Walt had more and more to say to George about how the organization should be managed. It took Walt only a matter of days to get beyond the generalized management techniques like budgeting and appraisal and begin to offer specific advice on the management of the physical therapy department.

Quickly George came to realize that he could virtually count on Walt to offer some criticism of most of his actions in running the department and most of administration's actions in running the hospital. George did not appreciate this turn in his relationship with an otherwise good employee. George had always seen Walt as an excellent performer as a physical therapist, perhaps somewhat opinionated but not to any harmful extent. Recently, however, he had come to regard Walt as an ongoing critical presence who was monitoring his every move as a manager, and as a result something of a nuisance.

The deteriorating situation came to a head one day when Walt attempted to intercede in a squabble between two other physical therapy employees and, when George entered the situation, proceeded to criticize George's handling of the matter in front of the other employees.

George immediately took Walt into his office for a private one-on-one conversation. He first told Walt that although he was free to offer his suggestions, opinions, and criticisms regarding management, he was never again to do so in the presence of others in the department. George then asked Walt, "It seems that lately you have had a great deal to say about management and specifically about how I manage this department. Why this sudden active interest in management?"

Walt answered, "In my physical therapy program we never learned a great deal about managing, you know, about running a department and getting people to do the work. So when I got interested in some of the things I saw you were involved in, I went looking for more education. Last month I finished the first course in a management program, a course called Introduction to Management Theory. Now I'm in the second course, called Supervisory Practice. I know what I'm hearing—and quite honestly, most of it's pretty simple stuff—and when I see things that I know aren't being handled right, I feel I have an obligation to this hospital to speak up."

George ended the discussion by again telling Walt that he expected all such criticism and advice to be offered in private and never again in front of other employees. Overall, the conversation did not go well; more than once George felt that Walt's remarks were edging toward insubordination. Because of the uneasy feeling the discussion left with him, George requested a meeting with Carl Miller, the hospital's vice president for human resources.

After describing the state of the relationship between him and Walt in some detail, George spread his hands in a gesture of helplessness and said to Carl, "I'm looking for your advice. Apparently on the strength of a course or two of textbook management, this guy suddenly has all the answers. What can I do with him?"

Questions:

1. If Walt continues to act as though he has all the answers, what can George do to encourage modification of this attitude? Explain your answer in detail.

2. If you were in Walt's position, how do you believe you should proceed in applying your newly acquired knowledge of management? Explain your answer and provide one or two illustrative examples.

3. What are the possible reasons behind George's growing aggravation with Walt, both the obvious and not-so-obvious? List a few possible reasons and comment on the validity of each.

CASE 11

Topic emphasis:	Delegation
Additional topics:	Management style
	Leadership
	Professional behavior

THE BUSY, BUSY MANAGER FINALLY DELEGATES

Director of materials management Don Weston was responsible for activities divided among five subordinate managers, some of whom themselves had subordinate supervisors. As someone responsible for a wide range of activities and many tasks, Don had always espoused a belief in active delegation of authority and active participative management as far as his five direct-reporting managers were concerned.

It seemed to Don as though a common response throughout the hospital to many problems and questions that arose was, "That's Don Weston's responsibility." In a way it made him feel good to be identified so strongly with many important activities.

Among Don's many responsibilities was membership, on behalf of the hospital, on several product committees of the region's group purchasing program. He also served on at least four hospital committees, including the product evaluation committee and the safety committee.

As is often the case with a growing health care institution and with the expanding field of health care itself, Don's job continued to grow until it reached a point at which he became painfully aware that he could no longer cover all of the bases as he had been doing for so long. He was missing committee meetings and failing to completely fulfill a number of his other responsibilities.

In an attempt to gain some relief, Don delegated representation on several committees to some of his subordinate managers and likewise delegated some other tasks that he had become too busy to handle. He thought that doing so would be wise for both him and his subordinate managers, so he was surprised to discover that his five managers were resentful of their newly delegated assignments. He inadvertently heard one manager say to another something about "Weston dumping off his responsibilities on us." Another, purchasing manager Ben Archer, said to Don directly, "Of all things, why did you have to stick me with the safety committee? Couldn't you take it any more?"

Questions:

1. What in the brief description of Don's role in the hospital suggests that the seeds for resistance to his delegation may have been long present? Explain in detail.

2. Identify and describe Don's primary failings in his working relationship with his subordinate managers.

3. Having met with resistance from his subordinate managers, how might Don address the matter of proper delegation so they might better appreciate the value of the tasks being delegated? In other words, what could Don be doing to help motivate his subordinate managers to willingly accept their delegated tasks?

CASE 12

Topic emphasis:	Change management
Additional topics:	Management style
	Decision-making
	Professionalism

PAID TO MAKE DECISIONS

Sherry Davis, a registered nurse with more than 10 years of management experience, was hired from outside as nursing director of the emergency division of City Hospital. It was Sherry's style to gain insight into how to manage a given operation by putting herself where the action was and becoming immersed in the work. However, she quickly discovered that her tendency to become deeply involved in the hands-on work drew reactions from staff members ranging from surprise to resentment. She also discovered that her predecessor, who had been in the position for several years, had been surreptitiously referred to as "The Friendly Ghost"—friendly because she usually seemed to be just that, and ghost because she was seen only rarely and fleetingly.

In spite of the legacy of "The Friendly Ghost," Sherry provided a certain management presence and seemed determined to remain deeply involved in the work of the department. She was also determined to significantly improve the level of professionalism in the department, a quality that had struck her from the first as decidedly lacking.

In a short time Sherry had moved to reinstate and reinforce a long-ignored dress code for the department, to eliminate personal telephone calls during working hours except for emergency situations, to curb chronic tardiness on the part of some staff members, to bar food and drink and reading material from working areas (also a reemphasis of long-ignored rules), and to curb the practice of changing scheduled days of work after the time limit allowed by department policy.

Sherry found her efforts frustrated at every turn. As she said to her immediate superior, "I can't understand the reaction. All I've done is insist that a few hospital rules be followed—mostly rules that have been there all along but were mostly ignored—and added a few twists unique to the emergency department. Just that, and yet the bitterness and lack of support and even resentment are so strong I could slice them. I'm getting all-out resistance from a few people I would still have to describe as good, professional nurses at heart."

Sherry's boss, the vice president for nursing service, said, "Do you suppose you might be pushing too hard, hitting them with one surprise after another without knowing how they felt and without asking for their cooperation?"

"That's possible," answered Sherry, "but now I'm committed on several fronts and I can't back down on any of them without looking bad to the department."

"Don't think of this as a contest of wills, or as some deadly game where compromise has no place. It may be necessary for you to back down temporarily in some areas or at least to hold a few of your improvements up in the air for a while. It may not hurt to fall back and involve a few of your staff in looking at the apparent needs of the department."

With a touch of impatience Sherry said, "Oh, I've heard all the textbook stuff about participative management. That may be the way for some, but that's never been my style. I'm paid to make decisions so I make them. I don't try to avoid responsibility by encouraging employees to make my decisions, and I don't try to curry favor with the staff by asking for their advice about every little thing that comes up."

Questions:

1. Identify and describe the weaknesses, if any are apparent, in Sherry's statement, "I don't try to avoid responsibility by encouraging employees to make my decisions." What, if anything, has Sherry overlooked?

2. What has essentially been wrong with Sherry's approach to raising the level of professionalism in the department? Why has it been wrong?

3. Ideally, how should Sherry have initially approached her plan to improve the emergency department?

4. Given the state of affairs Sherry is faced with in light of her conversation with the nursing vice president, how should she go about attempting to salvage some of her ideas and proceed with the improvement of the department? Keep in mind that at this stage her actions have probably had serious effects on her chances of implementing her plans.

CASE 13

Topic emphasis: Change management

Additional topics: Communication
                          Leadership
                          Motivation

THE PROMOTION

With more than adequate advance notice, Memorial Hospital's director of health information management (HIM) resigned to take a similar position with a hospital in another state. Within the department it was assumed that Eunice Jamison, the department's assistant director and a registered record administrator (R.R.A.) whom most staff thought was being groomed as the director's eventual replacement, would be appointed director. However, a month after the former director's departure the department was still operating without a designated director. Day-to-day operations had apparently been left in Eunice's hands ("apparently," because nothing had been said to her), but the hospital's chief operating officer, normally the HIM director's immediate superior, had begun to make some of the administrative decisions affecting HIM.

After another month had passed Eunice learned "through the grapevine" that the hospital had interviewed several candidates for the position of director of HIM. However, nobody had been hired.

During the next several weeks Eunice tried several times to discuss her uncertain status with the chief operating officer. Each time she was put off; once she was told simply to "keep on doing what you're now doing."

Four months after the former director's departure Eunice was promoted to director of health information management. The first instruction she received from the chief operating officer was to abolish the position of assistant director.

Questions:

1. Would the employees' view of Eunice when she was finally promoted likely be the same as it would have been if she had been promoted immediately following the former director's departure? Fully explain why or why not.

2. What effects, if any, could the delay have on the new director's ability to effectively fill the position of department director?

CASE 14

Topic emphasis:	People problems
Additional topics:	Communication
	Decision-making
	Professional behavior

THE VOICE

Sally Comstock was nurse manager of a medical/surgical unit at Memorial Hospital. One evening as she sat working on schedules at the nurses' station well after her "normal" work day had ended, a physician with whom she had had a number of confrontations strode up to the station bearing a stormy look. He said, "I want that nurse of yours, that Margo what's-her-face, kept out of Mr. Wilson's room. And that's final, no arguments."

Sally politely asked, "Do you mean Margo Adams?" Sally knew very well that was whom the doctor was talking about.

"Whatever, the only Margo on your staff. She's got my patient so upset that his blood pressure's elevated."

"What's the problem?"

"Her voice! Her loud, screechy, irritating voice. Even something simple like 'Lift your hand, please,' comes out like a shrill command. She's in the room two minutes and my patient is ready to climb the walls." (Sally thought: And apparently you, too, doctor, are ready to climb the walls.)

Sally responded, "Doctor, right now, in addition to me—and I'm supposed to have gone home long ago—there are only two R.N.s to cover this whole unit on the second shift. And Mrs. Adams—an extremely capable nurse, by the way—is one of the two. We've been understaffed for months, and I don't see things getting any better in the near future. I don't know what I can do about Margo or her voice."

"*I* know what you can do about her," the doctor countered. "You can do exactly as I say and keep her out of Mr. Wilson's room. And if she so much as steps through the door of that room again I'm going to enter that fact on the patient's chart and make it a medical order that she be kept away from him."

The doctor stormed away, leaving Sally to ponder the problem of Margo Adams's voice.

Instructions:

Develop one or more potential solutions, attempting to equally accommodate, as far as possible:

1. The needs of the patient.
2. The demands of the physician (to whatever extent you believe them to be justified).
3. The staffing requirements of the unit.

CASE 15

Topic emphasis:	Management authority
Additional topics:	Change management
	Delegation
	Decision-making
	People problems
	Professional behavior

WHEN PUSH COMES TO SHOVE,
THE BOSS IS ALWAYS THE BOSS

Charles Mason is controller of Morgan General Hospital. He reports to Robert Green, vice president for finance. Robert has been with the hospital for a number of years, having started as a staff accountant and worked his way up through controller and eventually into the top finance position, which he has held for about five years.

Charles is the third controller reporting to Robert in less than five years. He has never heard a predecessor's opinion of Robert, but his own is that Robert does not practice delegation to any significant extent and attempts to hang onto as much as possible of the running of the departments under his control.

Recently Morgan General entered a period of rapid and extensive change. The adoption of a new accounting system, accompanied by expanded computerization, changed the workload requirements in accounting. The data processing section under Charles grew in size, but general accounting and patient accounting found themselves overstaffed for their current needs.

Charles accepted the eventual necessity of reducing the manpower in the accounting sections; however, the new budget year was coming up and he had not yet been able to achieve reduction through normal attrition as had been his goal. It looked likely that he would have to make at least two cuts by layoff. If someone were to retire that would avoid a layoff, but Charles knew of no one who was planning to leave in the foreseeable future. The only person close to retirement was Ned Kline of patient accounting. Ned was a few months short of age 62, but he had expressed his intention to work until age 65.

Along with Charles's manpower budget projections, Robert requested Charles's plans for bringing his staff down to the required level. Charles submitted two names for layoff—Norm Brown of general accounting and Ralph Miller of patient accounting. Robert responded by suggesting that Charles get rid of Ned and Jerry Victor, who was also in patient accounting.

Charles did not agree, and he asked for Robert's reasons. Robert responded that Jerry and Ned were the two least productive individuals in the department and that Ned, in addition to being marginally productive, had a chronic attitude problem. Charles disputed both of these suggested actions. In his own recommendations he had gone by straight seniority, although he was not required to do so. He simply felt that seniority, if applied consistently, was the most defensible way of approaching reduction in staff. Charles considered Jerry capable, and Jerry was third from the bottom in seniority. Norm and Ralph were the logical choices to go on a last-in, first-out basis. In general, Charles agreed with Robert about Ned's productivity and attitude, but he felt that keeping such a person around for some 15 years had been a management mistake and it would not be fair to get rid of the man this close to retirement.

Robert told Charles to do what he felt was right; he was only making suggestions.

Charles knew there was no love lost between Robert and Jerry; they had occasional differences on business matters, and when they communicated at all it was briefly and curtly. Charles felt that Robert was using this opportunity to weed out people he did not particularly like.

One week later Robert and Charles were again face-to-face on the same issue. Robert asked if Charles had revised his recommendations. The layoffs were to take place in stages, with a pay period between individual layoffs. One employee from accounting had to go at the end of the current week. Charles indicated that his first choice to go was Norm.

Robert reminded Charles of his earlier recommendations. He still felt that Ned and Jerry should go. He pointed out that Ned would not be hurt because he had a fair amount in the contributory retirement plan and was also known to own some rental property on the side. He suggested that it did not matter that Ned wanted to keep working.

On Wednesday, two days prior to the target for the first layoff, Charles prepared the termination notice for Norm. He went to Robert for the necessary higher-management signature. Robert refused to sign the notice. Robert said to Charles, "What would you do if I gave you a direct order to lay off Jerry and Ned?"

Charles answered, "I don't know. I might refuse, or I might not."

Robert said he was going to keep the notice for a while and do some thinking. Charles went away pondering what he considered to be the basic unfairness of Robert's actions and wondering what he would do if it came to a confrontation.

The next day, Thursday, Robert again sent for Charles. He had not signed the termination notice for Norm. Instead, before him he had termination notices for Jerry and Ned, the latter dated for one pay period following the former. Robert had already signed them. He showed the notices to Charles and said, "I feel it's in the best interests of the finance division and the institution as a whole if these are the two people who leave. It's my belief that they are the least capable employees in the finance division. I'm sorry you chose to ignore my suggestions, and now I have to put them in the form of a direct order. You will put these two employees on layoff. Sign these notices and have them delivered and talk to the people as necessary."

Instructions:

Consider the primary alternatives open to Charles. He may either (a) follow Robert's instructions and lay off Jerry and Ned, or (b) refuse to do so and risk the consequences. Fully explore arguments both for and against each alternative, citing any assumptions you feel are necessary and describing circumstances that might mitigate a decision one way or the other.

CASE 16

Topic emphasis:	Management authority
Additional topics:	Communication
	Criticism and discipline
	Decision-making
	Professional behavior

LOOKING FOR THE LIMITS

When licensed professional engineer (P.E.) Bill Cable accepted the position of manager of engineering and maintenance at County Hospital, his immediate superior, chief operating officer Peter Jackson, told him that he would not find a great deal of decision-making guidance written out in policy and procedure form. As Peter expressed it, "Common sense is the overriding policy." However, Peter cautioned Bill about the necessity to see him about matters involving employee discipline, because the hospital was especially sensitive to union overtures in the service and maintenance areas.

Early during Bill's third week on the job a matter arose that seemed to him to call for disciplinary action of a routine nature. Remembering Peter's precaution, he tried to see the chief operating officer several times over a period of three days. Being unable to get to Peter and receiving no response to his messages specifically describing the situation, Bill went ahead and took action rather than risk losing credibility through procrastination. When he was finally able to obtain an audience with Peter some several days later, Bill described the situation and the action he had taken. Peter agreed with Bill, and of Bill's apparent concern for getting to him quickly he said, "What's the big deal? As I said, common sense is the best policy, and yours was a sound, common-sense decision."

When a similar situation arose some weeks later and again Bill could not get directly to Peter despite several tries, once again he took action. However, this time the disciplinary action involved an employee whom Bill later learned was a vocal informal leader of a sizeable group of discontented employees. The disciplinary action blew up in Bill's face and provided the active union organizers with an issue that they instantly took up as a rallying point.

Peter was furious with Bill, accusing him of deliberately overstepping his authority by refusing to bring such problems to his attention as he had directed.

Instructions:

1. Fully explain how Bill might go about determining the true limits of his decision-making authority.

2. The limits of an individual manager's authority are ultimately those limits established by the manager's immediate superior—in Bill's case, Peter. Outline a possible approach for getting Peter to help Bill define the actual limits of his authority.

CASE 17

Topic emphasis:	Management authority
Additional topics:	Communication
	Leadership
	People problems
	Professional behavior

BREACH OF CONFIDENCE

Mary French is nurse manager of a medical/surgical unit. Her close friend, June Ross, is nurse manager of a similar unit located on the floor directly above Mary's unit.

One day following their normal shift, an obviously troubled June sought Mary's advice as both a nurse manager and a friend relative to a delicate situation existing in June's unit. Mary and June held a lengthy conversation in a private corner of the nurses' lounge. June asked Mary to keep the matter confidential.

Their conversation was observed, but not heard, by their immediate supervisor, assistant nursing director Peg Jenkins. The following morning Peg visited Mary in her unit and said, "I saw you talking with June yesterday. I've gotten a growing sense that something is wrong on her floor, and I think it's gotten to a point where it's affecting the unit's performance. Please tell me about it."

Mary responded, "The matter is largely personal, and I would be violating a confidence if I told you."

Peg said, "Anything that affects nursing performance affects patient care whether it's personal or not. I want to be told. Now."

Instructions:

1. In not more than two or three sentences, draft a simple response that Mary could consider delivering to Peg then and there. Provide a rationale for this immediate response.

2. Describe the steps that you believe Mary should take if her supervisor is not satisfied with a "simple response" and refuses to let the matter rest.

CASE 18

Topic emphasis:	Delegation
Additional topics:	Management style
	Professional behavior

THE GIVER OF ORDERS

Nurse manager Mary Bennett was not certain whether she had a real problem with charge nurse Kelly Johnson. She described the situation over coffee with human resources director Jane Arnold: "I appointed Kelly Johnson as charge nurse to cover my days off. She had never worked in a charge capacity before and I really didn't know much about her work or her capability, but she was recommended by my predecessor. I went along with the recommendation and appointed Kelly because I was new to the hospital and hardly knew anything about anyone."

Jane smiled. "Kelly hasn't worked out?"

"I don't know, but something isn't right. I've had a number of complaints from staff to the effect that whenever I'm not there—that is, when Kelly's in charge—she delegates everything to the others, even to the point of handing out jobs that I specifically asked her to take care of. As I see it, the things that I do when I'm here are the things that Kelly should be doing when she's in charge in my place. But she delegates everything, and I've been told that the others are running their feet off while she sips coffee and pushes papers."

Jane said, "Do you suppose that a lot of the things she delegates really should be delegated? I mean, if she's really going to learn how to manage, shouldn't she be delegating?'

Mary answered, "I don't know much about management theory, like what you should or shouldn't do when you delegate and all that, but I do know that the object of delegation isn't to hand out all of your work so you have nothing left to do. Kelly's a good staff nurse, at least when I'm around to see her working in that capacity. But she's probably on the wrong track if she thinks that being a charge nurse entitles her to be a full-time giver of orders."

Instructions:

1. Identify and explain the possible problems and weaknesses in Mary's concept of delegation, and her approach to delegation.

2. Do the same for Kelly, thus providing the basis for comparing their apparently differing beliefs about the nature and practice of delegation.

3. Recommend an approach for Mary to consider trying in an effort to get the situation with the charge nurse onto a track toward improvement.

CASE 19

Topic emphasis:	Delegation
Additional topics:	Leadership
	Management style
	Personal effectiveness

TAKE YOUR CHOICE

Imagine that you are a registered nurse with some 20 years' experience, and you have spent half of that time as nursing director of a small (65-bed) rural hospital. You recently applied for the position of assistant director of nursing service at a 375-bed city hospital. During your initial interview, the nursing director posed four sets of "conditions" and asked you to state which of these best described the circumstances under which you believed such a position should be taken. The "conditions" were as follows:

1. You step into the job with the full responsibility and authority of the position as experienced by your predecessor.

2. You assume the full authority of the position but have somewhat reduced responsibility because of your newness to the job.

3. You have equal responsibility and authority but at a lesser level than your predecessor, leaving you room to "grow" into the position.

4. You assume the full responsibility of the position but are permitted to exercise less authority than your predecessor (again, because you are "new").

Instructions:

1. Fully describe the advantages and disadvantages of each set of "conditions" relative to (a) yourself and (b) the institution.

2. Decide under which set or sets of "conditions" you would consider taking the job, and explain why you would choose thusly.

CASE 20

Topic emphasis:	Professional behavior
Additional topics:	Delegation
	Management style
	People problems

THE INEFFECTIVE SUBORDINATE

Assistant nursing director Kate Dyer was finally forced to admit—at least to herself—that she was going nowhere in her long-running attempt to get nurse manager Susan Foster to behave as a manager ought to behave. Summarizing the recent occasions on which Susan and her performance had come to Kate's attention, Kate came up with the following list:

*   Whenever Kate went through Susan's unit, she found Susan's desk in disarray and found Susan herself invariably behind in her work.

*   Susan seemed to experience a great deal of difficulty in making important meetings. In fact, she had missed three of the last four nurse manager meetings, and she didn't even show up at the fourth meeting until it was half over.

*   Kate's specific suggestions as to tasks that Susan might consider delegating to some of her subordinates have apparently been ignored.

*   Some weeks earlier Kate had asked Susan for a detailed written listing as to how the various nursing duties on her floor might be divided up among the unit's staff members. Susan did respond to the request.

In general, Susan seemed to have but two answers for many of the questions put to her by peers and supervisors alike. To questions that were general and nonthreatening, such as "How is everything going?" she would simply answer, "Just fine." However, if a question seemed intended to determine why something specific had not been done, Susan could be counted on to answer, with a pained expression on her face, "I simply haven't been able to get to it."

Instructions:

1. Although Susan's performance is obviously lacking in a number of ways, Kate might best begin by examining some elements of her own performance and her own leadership style. Identify the elements of the case description that might have prompted the foregoing statement calling for examination of Kate's style, and describe the implications of those elements concerning Kate's style and performance.

2. Identify the weakest elements of Kate's management style and explain why they are weak.

3. Assuming Kate is able to successfully address the deficiencies in her own approach to management, explain where and how she should begin in trying to determine whether Susan has the potential to become a truly effective nurse manager.

Index